SPSS in Practice

An illustrated guide

2nd Edition

Basant K. Puri MA, MB BChir, MRCPsych, DipMath, BSc (Hons) MathSci, DipStat, PhD
Consultant & Senior Lecturer, MRI Unit, MRC Clinical Sciences Centre,
Imperial College School of Medicine, Hammersmith Hospital, London; Honorary Consultant in Imaging,
Department of Radiology, Hammersmith Hospital, London, UK

ARNOLD

A member of the Hodder Headline Group
LONDON • NEW YORK • NEW DELHI

First published in Great Britain in 1996 as *Statistics in Practice* by
Arnold, a member of the Hodder Headline Group,
338 Euston Road, London NW1 3BH

Second edition published in 2002

http://www.arnoldpublishers.com

Distributed in the USA by
Oxford University Press Inc.,
198 Madison Avenue, New York, NY10016
Oxford is a registered trademark of Oxford University Press

Whilst the advice and information in this book are believed to be true and
accurate at the date of going to press, neither the author nor the publisher
can accept any legal responsibility or liability for any errors or omissions
that may be made. In particular (but without limiting the generality of the
preceding disclaimer) every effort has been made to check drug dosages;
however, it is still possible that errors have been missed. Furthermore,
dosage schedules are constantly being revised and new side-effects
recognized. For these reasons the reader is strongly urged to consult the
drug companies' printed instructions before administering any of the drugs
recommended in this book.

British Library Cataloguing in Publication Data
A catalogue record for this book is available from the British Library

Library of Congress Cataloguing-in-Publication Data
A catalogue record for this book is available from the Library of Congress

ISBN 0 340 76112 1

1 2 3 4 5 6 7 8 9 10

Publisher: Georgina Bentliff
Development Editor: Heather Smith
Production Editor: James Rabson
Production Controller: Martin Kerans
Cover Design: Terry Griffiths

Typeset in 10 on 13 pt Sabon by Phoenix Photosetting, Chatham, Kent
Printed and bound in Malta by Gutenberg Press Ltd

What do you think about this book? Or any other Arnold title?
Please send your comments to feedback.arnold@hodder.co.uk

C O N T E N T S

1006255576 ⸗

PREFACE

The release of the 10th version of SPSS has necessitated the writing of a new edition of this book, owing to the fact that SPSS version 10 differs significantly from its predecessors. The production of the second edition of the book has afforded me the opportunity to rewrite most chapters, not only to bring the procedures and illustrations in line with the new version of SPSS, but also to expand and clarify certain topics, such as the editing of graphical output and the nature and interpretation of analysis of variance output tables. Once again, liberal use has been made of actual screen shots from the monitor of a personal computer running the statistical tests described. Also, in this edition the data sets that are shipped with this software package have been used to provide many of the practical examples described. These features of the book should enable the reader to find it relatively easy to master the use of many important and powerful tests that SPSS offers.

Basant K. Puri
Cambridge, England
2002

PREFACE TO THE
FIRST EDITION

This book offers a practical guide to using SPSS for Windows. Details are given of how to choose, access and use a variety of statistical procedures and charts available in this powerful statistics package. Rather than doing this by giving lists of commands, screen shots corresponding to what the user actually sees on the computer monitor have been used.

I should like to thank SPSS for giving me permission to reproduce screen shots from their software.

chapter 1

INTRODUCTION

AIMS OF THIS BOOK

This book provides a practical guide to using a popular statistical software package, SPSS for Windows. To this end, pictures are provided of the screen as you would see it if running version 10 (SPSS Inc., 2000).

The book considers the following aspects of the use of SPSS:

- data entry
- the choice of an appropriate statistical test
- exploring the data
- data transformation
- running statistical tests and producing graphical (chart) images.

In general, details of the theory underlying the statistical tests described are not provided; these are available in standard textbooks. Therefore, mathematical formulae and equations have generally been omitted.

BASIC CONCEPTS

DATA

The word data is the plural of datum, and is defined in the *Shorter Oxford English Dictionary* as:

> **Datum. Pl. data.** 1646. [L., neut. pa. pple. of *dare* give.] A thing given or granted; something known or assumed as fact, and made the basis of reasoning or calculation.

Many different fields of human endeavour, ranging from science and economics through to subjects in the humanities, give rise to data.

STATISTICS

Statistical techniques can be applied to carry out:

- data exploration
- summarizing data

- data analysis
- deriving inferences from data
- communication information
- decision making.

Before embarking on the application of the statistical techniques available in SPSS to a data set, it is always a good idea first to explore the data. This may include the use of graphical displays (available under the **Graph** menu of SPSS), as geometric representations of data are often much easier to understand than are results expressed solely in numerical form. Chapter 3 details some of the data exploration techniques available in SPSS.

VARIABLES

Definition
A variable is an observable quantity or attribute which varies from one member of the population being studied to another.

Classification

Figure 1.1 shows one way in which variables can be classified.

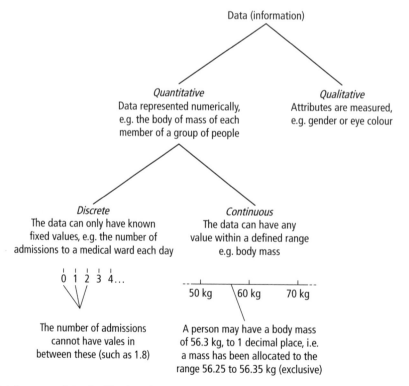

Figure 1.1 Summary of the classification of variables. Based on Puri BK (1996) *Statistics for the Health Sciences*, with permission from WB Saunders, London

Independent and dependent variables

The variable(s) whose values you wish to predict or summarize is(are) the dependent variable(s), while the variable(s) it(they) depend(s) on is(are) the independent variable(s). A dependent variable is also known as a response variable, while an independent variable is also known as an explanatory variable.

MEASUREMENT SCALES

There are four main types of measurement scale that can be used for different types of data: nominal, ordinal, interval and ratio. Their characteristics are summarized in Table 1.1.

Table 1.1 Types of measurement scale. Based on Puri BK (1996) *Statistics for the Health Sciences*, with permission from WB Saunders, London

Property	Nominal	Ordinal	Interval	Ratio
Categories mutually exclusive	✓	✓	✓	✓
Categories logically ordered		✓	✓	✓
Equal distance between adjacent categories			✓	✓
True zero point				✓

Nominal

A nominal measurement scale is a set of mutually exclusive categories that varies qualitatively but not quantitatively, for example gender and eye colour. For computational purposes, numbers are attached to these categories when using SPSS, but they do not imply that any one category is higher than another. For instance, when measuring eye colour, 1 may stand for blue, 2 for brown, 3 for green, and so on, but this does not imply that the categories are unequal.

Ordinal

An ordinal measurement scale differs from a nominal one in that the order among the original categories is preserved in the analysis; however, differences between adjacent categories are not equal. Examples include social class and the staging of cancer. Numbers attached to these categories reflect their relative order. For example, social class 1 is higher than social class 3; however, the difference between social classes 1 and 3 is not the same as the difference between social classes 3 and 5 (even though numerically $3 - 1 = 5 - 3$). In other words the numbers just give the rank.

The ordinal scale is more informative than the nominal scale. Variables measured on nominal and ordinal scales are discrete variables.

Interval

An interval scale differs from an ordinal one in that the differences between adjacent categories are equal; however, there is no true zero point. Examples include the

Fahrenheit and Celsius temperature scales. For example, 60 °C is a higher temperature than 50 °C, and the difference in temperature between 60 °C and 50 °C is the same as the difference between 30 °C and 20 °C; however, 60 °C is not twice the temperature of 30 °C, since 0 °C is not absolute zero.

The interval scale is more informative than nominal and ordinal scales.

Ratio

A ratio scale differs from an interval one in that there is a true zero point. Examples include the measurement of height in metres and the Kelvin temperature scale. For example, not only is the difference in height between 0.5 m and 0.4 m the same as the difference between 0.25 m and 0.15 m, but 0.5 m is twice 0.25 m.

The ratio scale is more informative than the preceding three scales. When using SPSS it is usually sufficient to class variables measured on both interval and ratio scales together as continuous variables.

PARAMETRIC AND NONPARAMETRIC TESTS

Parametric tests (such as the t-test and analysis of variance (ANOVA)) make a number of assumptions about the data being analyzed:

- the dependent variables are continuous (that is, they are measured on an interval or ratio scale)
- the underlying population from which the sample data are taken has a normal distribution
- when differences or measures of statistical association are being analyzed between two or more samples, the variances (or standard deviations) of these samples do not differ significantly.

On the other hand, nonparametric tests (such as the chi-square test and the Mann–Whitney U test) do not make such assumptions.

It is possible to test sample distributions for normality (see Chapter 4). If the distribution is not normal (that is, if it does not follow a normal distribution), then it may be possible to transform the data so that the transformed data are normal; the appropriate parametric statistical tests can then be applied to the transformed data. Data transformation is described in Chapter 5.

If continuous data do not follow a normal distribution and suitable data transformation is not possible, so that the data do not fulfil the assumptions of a parametric test, they can be converted into ordinal data and a nonparametric equivalent test can be used instead. However, in carrying out such a conversion there is a discarding of useful information from the data. Do bear in mind, however, that most parametric tests are usually robust to small deviations from the strict criteria outlined above.

If the assumptions of a parametric test *are* fulfilled, then conversion into ordinal data and the use of a nonparametric test results in a loss of statistical power. (The power of a hypothesis test is the probability that the null hypothesis is rejected when it is indeed false.)

USING MICROSOFT WINDOWS

It is assumed that the reader is familiar with the use of the Microsoft Windows environment. If not, you could work through the on-line **Getting Started** menu available in Windows. In Windows 2000 this is available from the **Help** menu of Windows (see Figure 1.2):

Start
    Help
        Contents
            Introducing Windows 2000 Professional
                Getting Started Book: Online Version
                    Windows 2000 Professional Getting Started

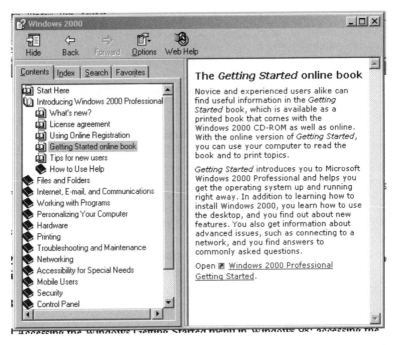

Figure 1.2 Accessing the Windows Getting Started menu in Windows 2000 after accessing the **Help** menu from the **Start** button

USING SPSS FOR WINDOWS

If the reader has not previously used this software, then it is recommended that the SPSS tutorial should be worked through first. This is usually available from the default dialogue box which opens when you first open SPSS version 10: choose the first option (**Run the tutorial**) as shown in Figure 1.3.

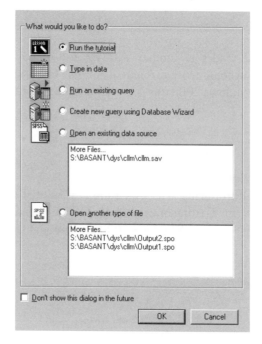

Figure 1.3 Accessing the SPSS tutorial in SPSS for Windows version 10 from the initial dialogue box

It can also be accessed using the following commands from within SPSS:

Help
> **Tutorial**

From now on, a command such as this will be denoted as

Help\Tutorial

Another very useful feature of SPSS is the Statistics Coach, which can be accessed by

Help\Coach

(These commands are also accessible from the keyboard; for example **Help\Coach** can be obtained by pressing **<SHIFT C>** at any time during an SPSS session.) The first window you see in the Statistics Coach is shown in Figure 1.4.

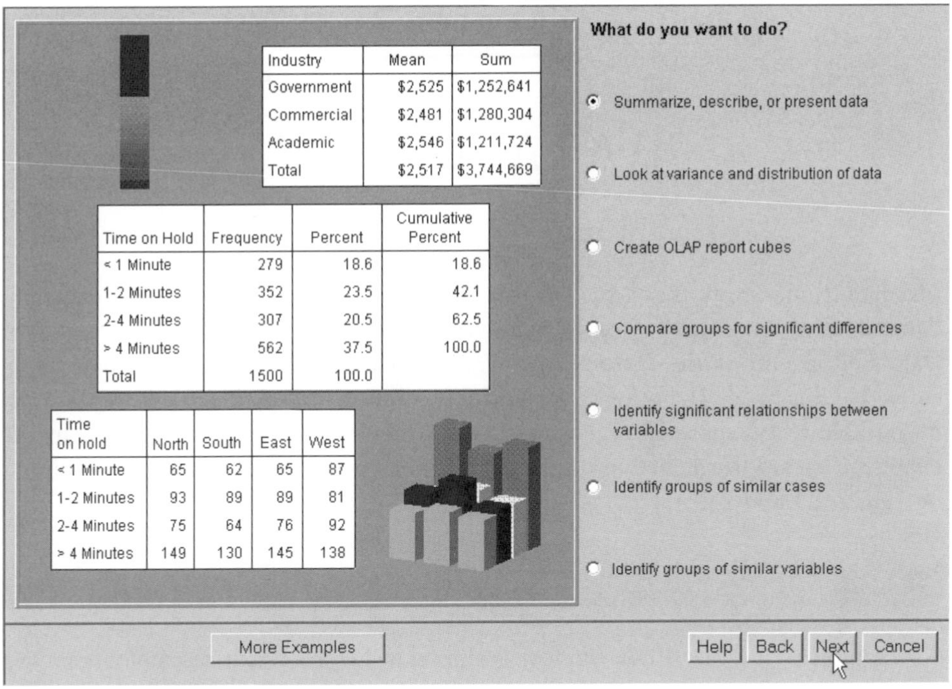

What do you want to do?

Industry	Mean	Sum
Government	$2,525	$1,252,641
Commercial	$2,481	$1,280,304
Academic	$2,546	$1,211,724
Total	$2,517	$3,744,669

○ Summarize, describe, or present data

○ Look at variance and distribution of data

Time on Hold	Frequency	Percent	Cumulative Percent
< 1 Minute	279	18.6	18.6
1-2 Minutes	352	23.5	42.1
2-4 Minutes	307	20.5	62.5
> 4 Minutes	562	37.5	100.0
Total	1500	100.0	

○ Create OLAP report cubes

○ Compare groups for significant differences

○ Identify significant relationships between variables

Time on hold	North	South	East	West
< 1 Minute	65	62	65	87
1-2 Minutes	93	89	89	81
2-4 Minutes	75	64	76	92
> 4 Minutes	149	130	145	138

○ Identify groups of similar cases

○ Identify groups of similar variables

More Examples

Help | Back | Next | Cancel

Figure 1.4 The first **Statistics Coach** box

chapter 2

DATA ENTRY

The data from a study, that is the information to be analyzed, are entered into an SPSS data file using the Data Editor. In SPSS version 10, there are two windows in SPSS Data Editor. One is the **Data View** window, which allows the actual data to be entered and viewed. The other is the **Variable View** window, which allows the *types* of variable to be specified and viewed. Both these windows are explained in this chapter. You can toggle between them by clicking on the appropriate tabs, as shown in Figures 2.1 and 2.2.

DATA VIEW

An example of a **Data View** window is shown in Figure 2.1. It resembles a spreadsheet in appearance.

	sex	race	region	happy	life	sibs	childs	age	educ	paeduc	maeduc	speduc	prestg
31	Female	White	North Eas	Pretty Happy	NAP	7	1	75	14	DK	8	NAP	66
32	Female	White	North Eas	Pretty Happy	NAP	0	3	58	16	12	DK	NAP	60
33	Male	White	North Eas	Pretty Happy	NAP	2	1	49	13	8	8	12	36
34	Male	White	North Eas	Very Happy	NAP	2	0	22	14	12	NA	NAP	49
35	Female	White	North Eas	Very Happy	Routine	0	3	44	17	18	12	20	52
36	Male	White	North Eas	Pretty Happy	NAP	1	2	48	19	15	NA	16	74
37	Female	White	North Eas	Not Too Happ	Routine	4	2	23	12	12	DK	12	4'
38	Male	White	North Eas	Very Happy	Exciting	1	0	56	15	NAP	DK	NAP	5'
39	Female	White	North Eas	Pretty Happy	NAP	5	0	25	13	8	DK	NAP	39
40	Female	White	West	Pretty Happy	Routine	2	0	78	12	NA	NA	NAP	45
41	Female	White	West	Pretty Happy	Exciting	3	3	37	15	13	14	12	46
42	Male	White	West	Very Happy	NAP	10	4	60	12	8	DK	12	36
43	Female	White	West	Very Happy	Routine	1	0	30	16	16	16	NAP	46
44	Male	White	West	Pretty Happy	NAP	1	0	21	13	NAP	14	NAP	50
45	Female	White	West	Very Happy	Exciting	0	3	65	13	NA	NA	NAP	DK,NA
46	Male	Other	West	Pretty Happy	Routine	2	Eight or	64	11	6	6	12	30
47	Male	White	West	Pretty Happy	NAP	6	0	31	18	14	11	16	64
48	Female	White	West	Pretty Happy	Routine	2	3	64	12	8	8	13	40
49	Male	White	West	Very Happy	Exciting	1	2	39	18	12	13	16	60
50	Female	White	West	Pretty Happy	Dull	1	0	29	16	16	12	NAP	46
51	Female	White	West	Not Too Happ	Routine	5	2	57	18	16	18	NAP	DK,NA
52	Male	White	West	Pretty Happy	NAP	1	0	35	14	12	DK	12	44
53	Male	Black	West	Not Too Happ	Exciting	8	0	22	15	12	16	NAP	2
54	Male	White	West	Very Happy	Exciting	3	0	35	16	12	12	NAP	5'
55	Male	White	West	Pretty Happy	Exciting	4	0	43	20	16	18	NAP	64
56	Female	White	West	Very Happy	Exciting	3	2	35	12	12	13	NAP	48
57	Female	White	West	Pretty Happy	Exciting	2	3	70	12	12	8	NAP	20
58	Male	White	West	Not Too Happ	Routine	3	2	49	13	12	8	12	39
59	Female	Other	West	Pretty Happy	Routine	2	1	21	11	NAP	16	NAP	DK,NA
60	Female	White	West	Very Happy	NAP	12	2	34	12	12	12	12	45
61	Male	Other	West	Not Too Happ	Exciting	4	1	34	12	12	7	12	36

Figure 2.1 Tabs for the **Data View** and **Variable View** windows in the SPSS Data Editor (taken from the sample data file 1991 US General Social Survey provided with SPSS). **Data View** is highlighted

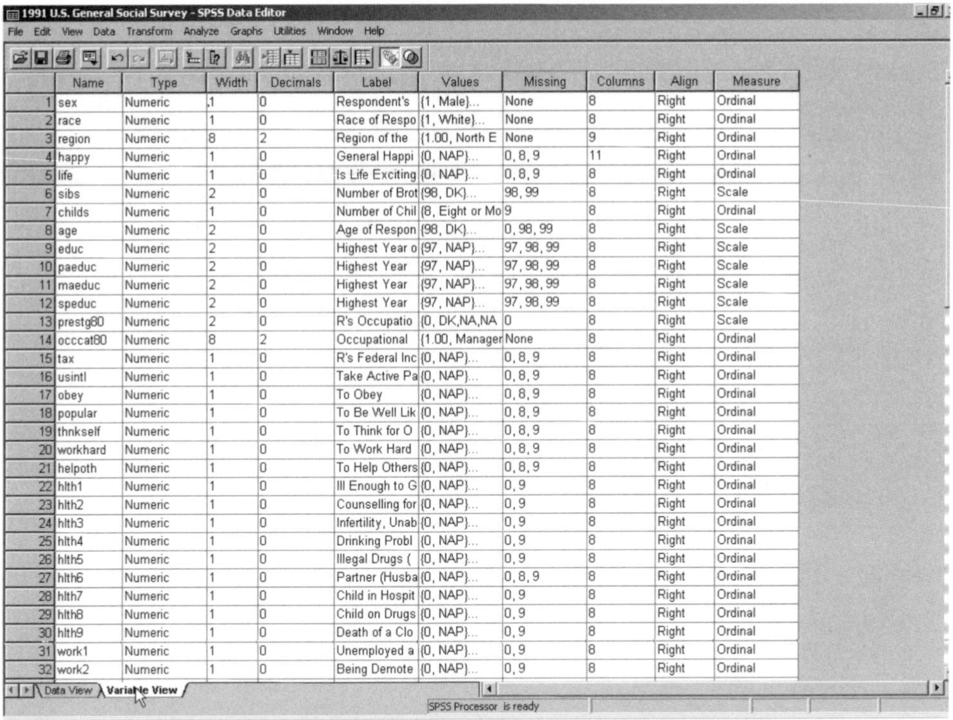

	Name	Type	Width	Decimals	Label	Values	Missing	Columns	Align	Measure
1	sex	Numeric	,1	0	Respondent's	{1, Male}...	None	8	Right	Ordinal
2	race	Numeric	1	0	Race of Respo	{1, White}...	None	8	Right	Ordinal
3	region	Numeric	8	2	Region of the	{1.00, North E	None	9	Right	Ordinal
4	happy	Numeric	1	0	General Happi	{0, NAP}...	0, 8, 9	11	Right	Ordinal
5	life	Numeric	1	0	Is Life Exciting	{0, NAP}...	0, 8, 9	8	Right	Ordinal
6	sibs	Numeric	2	0	Number of Brot	{98, DK}...	98, 99	8	Right	Scale
7	childs	Numeric	1	0	Number of Chil	{8, Eight or Mo	9	8	Right	Ordinal
8	age	Numeric	2	0	Age of Respon	{98, DK}...	0, 98, 99	8	Right	Scale
9	educ	Numeric	2	0	Highest Year o	{97, NAP}...	97, 98, 99	8	Right	Scale
10	paeduc	Numeric	2	0	Highest Year	{97, NAP}...	97, 98, 99	8	Right	Scale
11	maeduc	Numeric	2	0	Highest Year	{97, NAP}...	97, 98, 99	8	Right	Scale
12	speduc	Numeric	2	0	Highest Year	{97, NAP}...	97, 98, 99	8	Right	Scale
13	prestg80	Numeric	2	0	R's Occupatio	{0, DK,NA,NA	0	8	Right	Scale
14	occcat80	Numeric	8	2	Occupational	{1.00, Manager	None	8	Right	Ordinal
15	tax	Numeric	1	0	R's Federal Inc	{0, NAP}...	0, 8, 9	8	Right	Ordinal
16	usintl	Numeric	1	0	Take Active Pa	{0, NAP}...	0, 8, 9	8	Right	Ordinal
17	obey	Numeric	1	0	To Obey	{0, NAP}...	0, 8, 9	8	Right	Ordinal
18	popular	Numeric	1	0	To Be Well Lik	{0, NAP}...	0, 8, 9	8	Right	Ordinal
19	thnkself	Numeric	1	0	To Think for O	{0, NAP}...	0, 8, 9	8	Right	Ordinal
20	workhard	Numeric	1	0	To Work Hard	{0, NAP}...	0, 8, 9	8	Right	Ordinal
21	helpoth	Numeric	1	0	To Help Others	{0, NAP}...	0, 8, 9	8	Right	Ordinal
22	hlth1	Numeric	1	0	Ill Enough to G	{0, NAP}...	0, 9	8	Right	Ordinal
23	hlth2	Numeric	1	0	Counselling for	{0, NAP}...	0, 9	8	Right	Ordinal
24	hlth3	Numeric	1	0	Infertility, Unab	{0, NAP}...	0, 9	8	Right	Ordinal
25	hlth4	Numeric	1	0	Drinking Probl	{0, NAP}...	0, 9	8	Right	Ordinal
26	hlth5	Numeric	1	0	Illegal Drugs (	{0, NAP}...	0, 9	8	Right	Ordinal
27	hlth6	Numeric	1	0	Partner (Husba	{0, NAP}...	0, 8, 9	8	Right	Ordinal
28	hlth7	Numeric	1	0	Child in Hospit	{0, NAP}...	0, 9	8	Right	Ordinal
29	hlth8	Numeric	1	0	Child on Drugs	{0, NAP}...	0, 9	8	Right	Ordinal
30	hlth9	Numeric	1	0	Death of a Clo	{0, NAP}...	0, 9	8	Right	Ordinal
31	work1	Numeric	1	0	Unemployed a	{0, NAP}...	0, 9	8	Right	Ordinal
32	work2	Numeric	1	0	Being Demote	{0, NAP}...	0, 9	8	Right	Ordinal

Figure 2.2 Tabs for the **Data View** and **Variable View** windows in the SPSS Data Editor. **Variable View** is highlighted

ROWS

Each row represents a single case. In Figure 2.3, for example, the highlighted row represents the person detailed in row 2. From this row it can be seen that this person is a white female who at the time of data collection lived in the North East of the United States, was 'pretty happy', found life exciting, had two siblings and one child, was aged 32 years, and so on.

COLUMNS

Each column represents a single variable. In Figure 2.4, for example, the highlighted column represents the sex of the individuals.

CELLS

The value of each cell is determined by its row (case) and column (variable). In Figure 2.5, for example, the highlighted cell represents the sex (female) for the case in row number 2.

When you highlight a cell, a drop-down menu is offered (as shown by the appearance of the button with the downward arrow on the right-hand side of the cell in Figure 2.5). By clicking on the arrow, some potential values for the cell are made avail-

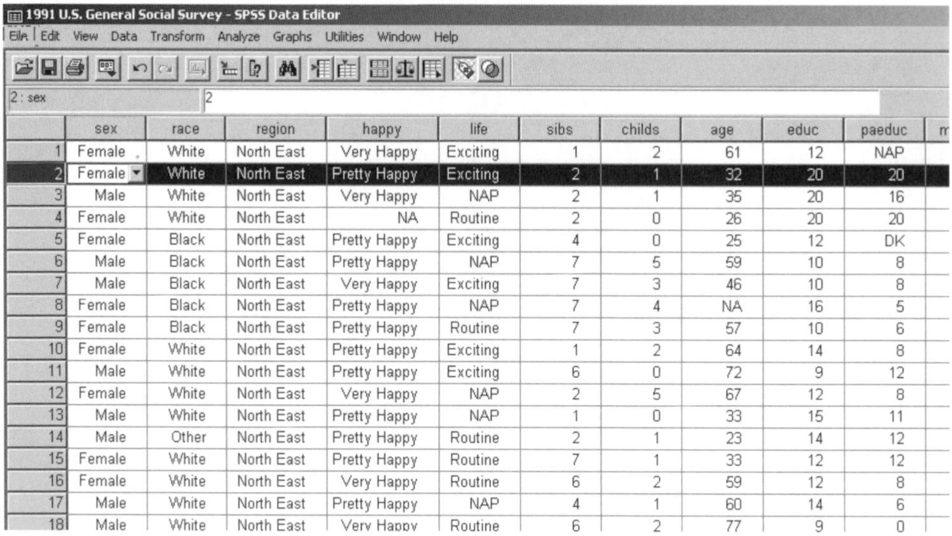

	sex	race	region	happy	life	sibs	childs	age	educ	paeduc
1	Female	White	North East	Very Happy	Exciting	1	2	61	12	NAP
2	Female	White	North East	Pretty Happy	Exciting	2	1	32	20	20
3	Male	White	North East	Very Happy	NAP	2	1	35	20	16
4	Female	White	North East	NA	Routine	2	0	26	20	20
5	Female	Black	North East	Pretty Happy	Exciting	4	0	25	12	DK
6	Male	Black	North East	Pretty Happy	NAP	7	5	59	10	8
7	Male	Black	North East	Very Happy	Exciting	7	3	46	10	8
8	Female	Black	North East	Pretty Happy	NAP	7	4	NA	16	5
9	Female	Black	North East	Pretty Happy	Routine	7	3	57	10	6
10	Female	White	North East	Pretty Happy	Exciting	1	2	64	14	8
11	Male	White	North East	Pretty Happy	Exciting	6	0	72	9	12
12	Female	White	North East	Very Happy	NAP	2	5	67	12	8
13	Male	White	North East	Pretty Happy	NAP	1	0	33	15	11
14	Male	Other	North East	Pretty Happy	Routine	2	1	23	14	12
15	Female	White	North East	Pretty Happy	Routine	7	1	33	12	12
16	Female	White	North East	Very Happy	Routine	6	2	59	12	8
17	Male	White	North East	Pretty Happy	NAP	4	1	60	14	6
18	Male	White	North East	Very Happy	Routine	6	2	77	9	0

Figure 2.3 A single case is represented by a row

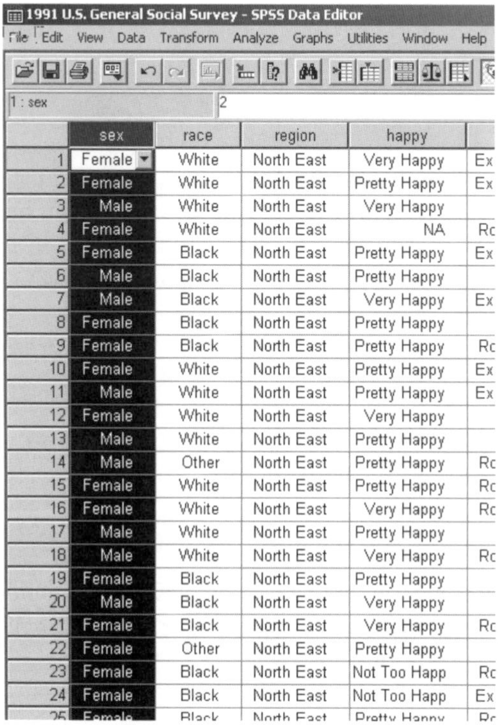

	sex	race	region	happy	
1	Female	White	North East	Very Happy	Ex
2	Female	White	North East	Pretty Happy	Ex
3	Male	White	North East	Very Happy	
4	Female	White	North East	NA	Rc
5	Female	Black	North East	Pretty Happy	Ex
6	Male	Black	North East	Pretty Happy	
7	Male	Black	North East	Very Happy	Ex
8	Female	Black	North East	Pretty Happy	
9	Female	Black	North East	Pretty Happy	Rc
10	Female	White	North East	Pretty Happy	Ex
11	Male	White	North East	Pretty Happy	Ex
12	Female	White	North East	Very Happy	
13	Male	White	North East	Pretty Happy	
14	Male	Other	North East	Pretty Happy	Rc
15	Female	White	North East	Pretty Happy	Rc
16	Female	White	North East	Very Happy	Rc
17	Male	White	North East	Pretty Happy	
18	Male	White	North East	Very Happy	Rc
19	Female	Black	North East	Pretty Happy	
20	Male	Black	North East	Very Happy	
21	Female	Black	North East	Very Happy	Rc
22	Female	Other	North East	Pretty Happy	
23	Female	Black	North East	Not Too Happ	Rc
24	Female	Black	North East	Not Too Happ	Ex
25	Female	Black	North East	Pretty Happy	Rc

Figure 2.4 A single variable is represented by a column

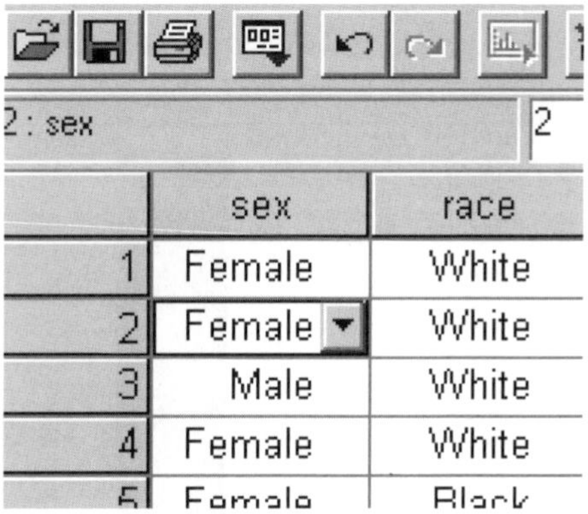

Figure 2.5 The value of a cell is determined by its row and column

able. For nominal and ordinal variables (see Chapter 1), all the potential values are available. For continuous (interval and ratio) variables, special values predefined by you in the **Variables View** window (see below) such as 'DK' for 'don't know', 'NA' for 'not applicable', etc., are available. In the case of the cell highlighted in Figure 2.5, since the corresponding variable, sex, refers to nominal data, all the possible options (in this case, male and female) are made available from the drop-down menu, as shown in Figure 2.6. By clicking on any of these options, that option is then inserted into the cell and replaces any existing value in that cell. This can be useful when entering data (see below) or editing data in **Data View**.

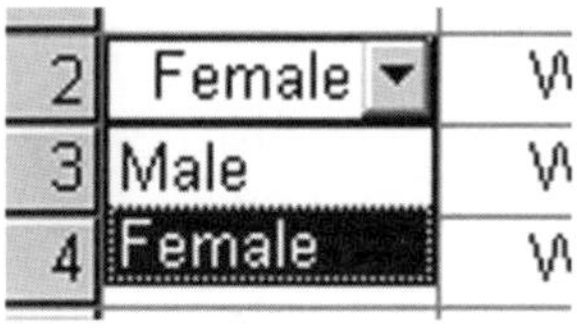

Figure 2.6 Variable values offered from the drop-down menu of a cell

Cells contain a period/full-stop when they are empty (Figure 2.7) or when they correspond to missing data (Figure 2.8).

ENTERING DATA

The actual data values are entered directly in **Data View** (in SPSS Data Editor). The variables are defined in **Variable View**.

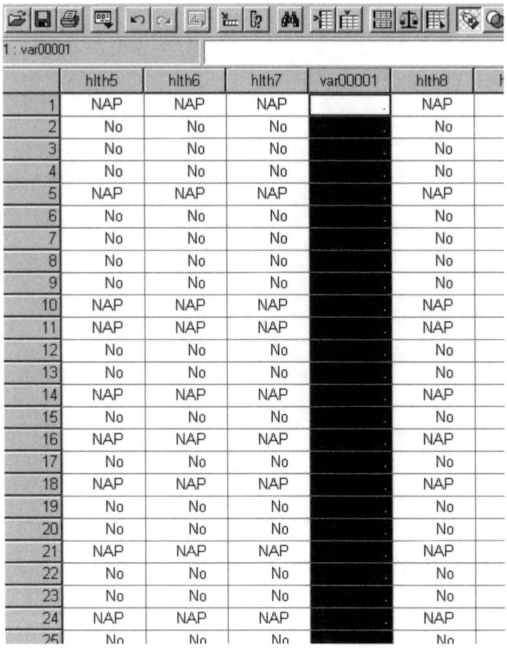

Figure 2.7 Empty cells (highlighted); the column is a new variable that has been inserted into the **Data View** window

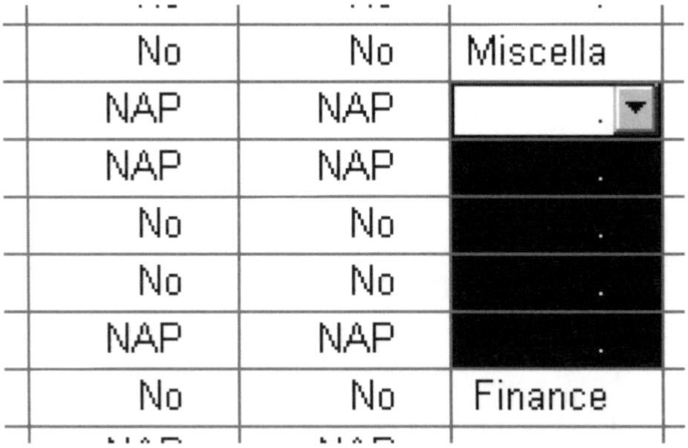

Figure 2.8 Cells with missing data cells (highlighted)

STANDARD NUMERICAL DATA

In SPSS, a numeric (numerical) variable refers to a variable whose values are displayed in standard numerical format, using the decimal point delimiter specified in Windows, for example 0.37. In this book the full stop is used to display a decimal point. In some countries a comma (,) is preferred. If you need to change your Windows setting for the way the decimal place is displayed, you can do so in **Control Panel\Regional Settings** in Windows.

As well as accepting numerical data in this standard format, data can be entered using Scientific Notation (see Figure 2.13 below) in which, for instance, $3.7E - 1 = 3.7 \times 10^{-1} = 0.37$. The SPSS default is to accept numerical data in standard format during data entry.

Numerical data are entered by selecting the appropriate cells (using the mouse or cursor keys) and typing in the required numbers. Each value appears in the cell editor (Figure 2.9) where it can be edited, if necessary, before entering.

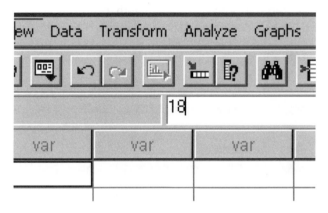

Figure 2.9 The cell editor

After pressing **<ENTER>** (or a cursor key) the data value is entered into the **Data View** spreadsheet, as shown in Figure 2.10. Note that if you have not defined the name of the variable, then SPSS gives it a unique name (in this case var00005). How to define a variable name is described in the next section.

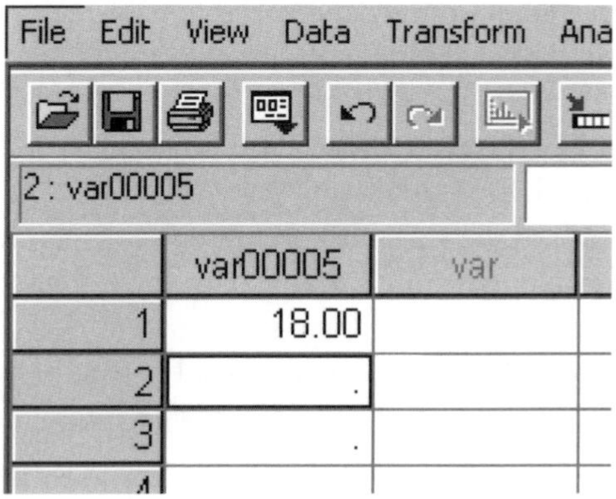

Figure 2.10 Entered data value with a default SPSS variable name

DEFINING VARIABLES

To enter non-numeric types of data, first the variable must be defined. You need to enter the **Variable View** window. Even if you are entering just numeric data (see previous section) you will still need to enter the **Variable View** window as you will probably wish at least to define your variable name. To enter **Variable View** you can either toggle between **Data View** and **Variable View** using the tab as shown in Figures 2.1 and 2.2, or else in **Data View** you can double click (with the left mouse button) the variable name at the head of the column.

Once you are in **Variable View**, you will see that this time each row corresponds to a variable. For example, for a new dataset relating to eye colour, the second row in **Variable View** in Figure 2.11 corresponds to the variable eye colour.

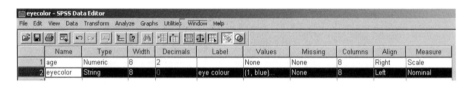

Figure 2.11 A single variable is represented by a row in **Variable View**

It is also clear from Figure 2.11 that as you go along each row in **Variable View** you can specify the following 10 characteristics of each variable:

1. Name – the variable name that you choose
2. Type – the variable type
3. Width – the width of the entries (the number of alphanumeric characters)
4. Decimals – the number of digits to the right of the decimal place for the entries (e.g. enter 2 for Decimals in order to input data such as 3.14, etc.)
5. Label – the variable label (if any); the variable name can only be a maximum of eight alphanumeric characters long, so you may need to specify a variable label in addition
6. Values – the value labels (see below)
7. Missing – the values (if any) of missing data
8. Columns – the width of the variable column to be displayed in **Data View**
9. Align – how you would like your variable data to be aligned in the corresponding column in **Data View**
10. Measure – the nature of the data for the variable (e.g. nominal, ordinal, or scale (i.e. continuous–interval or ratio)).

When you first enter a new variable, the above characteristics of the variable are given default values (e.g. Numeric for Type).

1. NAME

Highlight the cell in the first column of the variable row. Then simply type the name of the variable. You are limited to a maximum of eight alphanumeric characters (a, b, c, ..., y, z, A, B, C, ..., Y, Z, 0, 1, 2, ..., 9, _). While the underscore (_) character is allowed, hyphens (-), ampersands (&) and spaces are not allowed.

In Figure 2.11 you can see that the name used for the second variable is eyecolor.

2. TYPE

If you are not happy with the default data type given (usually numeric), highlight the cell in the second column of the variable row. You are offered a button with an ellipsis-like symbol (...). This is shown in Figure 2.12.

Figure 2.12 The result of highlighting a cell in the **Type** column in **Variable View**

Clicking on the button brings up the **Variable Type** dialogue box, as shown in Figure 2.13.

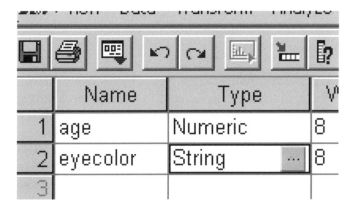

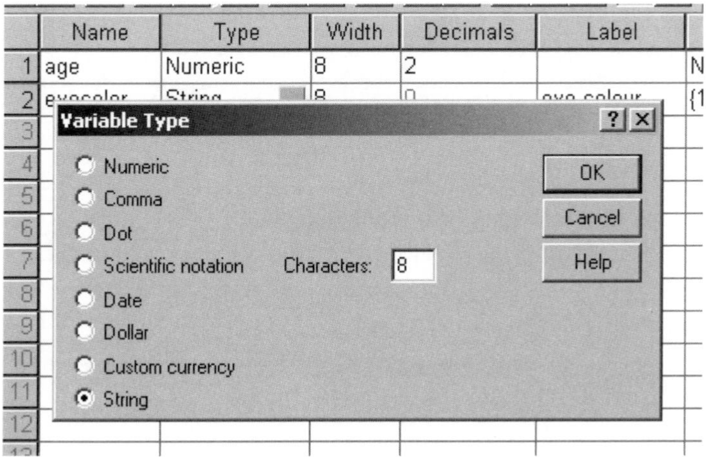

Figure 2.13 The **Variable Type** box

Simply choose the type of variable you wish by selecting the corresponding radio button. SPSS allows the entry of the following types of data:

- Numeric – numerical data in standard format (see above)
- Comma – a numerical variable in which values displayed with commas dividing every 3 places, and with a period as a decimal delimiter
- Dot – a numerical variable in which values displayed with periods dividing every 3 places, and with a comma as a decimal delimiter
- Scientific notation – see above
- Date – a number of formats are available for displaying dates (for example when entering dates of birth)
- Dollar
- Custom currency
- String – the values can contain any characters up to the length defined in the **Width** cell of the variable row in **Variable View**; upper and lower case letters are considered to be different.

You can alter the maximum number of characters for a string variable by altering the number in the box by **Characters**; in Figure 2.13 this is given as 8. Alternatively, you can alter this number back in **Variable View** by changing the number in the **Width** cell of the variable (see below).

By default, new variables are usually assigned as being numeric, with eight characters, including two digits to the right of the decimal place. This is shown in Figure 2.14. You can alter both the width and the number of digits to the right of the decimal place (**Decimal Places**) by altering the values in the corresponding windows in this box; in Figure 2.14 these default values are 8 and 2 respectively.

If your variable consists of dates (e.g. dates of birth or dates of testing) then when you choose **Date** in the **Variable Type** box (Figure 2.13) you are offered several

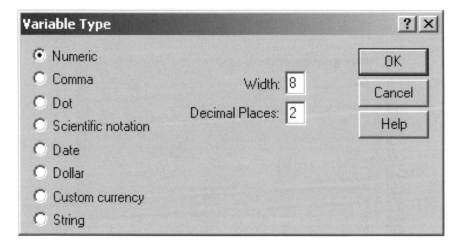

Figure 2.14 The usual default **Variable Type** box

choices for the date format. This will govern the way you enter the dates in **Data View**. For example, if you wish to enter the date 25 February 2005 in the form 25.02.2005, then make the selection highlighted in Figure 2.15.

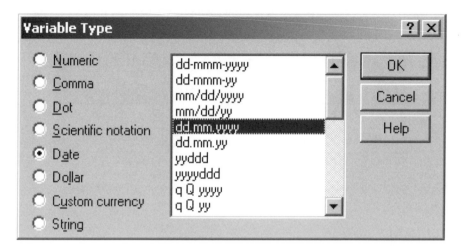

Figure 2.15 Choosing **Date** in the **Variable Type** box

3. WIDTH

This refers to the width of the actual data entries. The default width is usually given as 8. However, this may not be sufficient for your needs. For example, if one of your variables is a string variable consisting of the Christian names of subjects, then if you wish to store (and display) more than the first eight characters of each name, you will have to change the width setting.

If you are not happy with the default width given (usually 8), highlight the cell in the third column (headed **Width**) of the variable row in **Variable View** (Figure 2.11). Two small buttons appear in the right-hand side of the cell, as shown in Figure 2.16. The upper button has an up arrow on it, and the lower button a down arrow. You can increase the default value setting (in increments of one) by clicking on the up arrow.

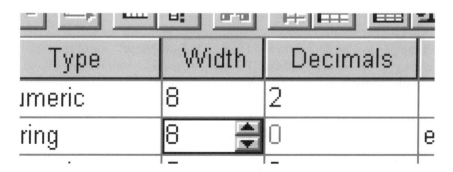

Figure 2.16 The result of highlighting a cell in the **Width** column in **Variable View**

Similarly, you can decrease the value (in decrements of one) by clicking on the down arrow. If you keep either button pressed down, then the value keeps increasing or decreasing automatically until you release the left mouse button.

Alternatively, you can select the default value by double-clicking on it, to highlight it as in Figure 2.17. Then type the new value, which replaces the previous one.

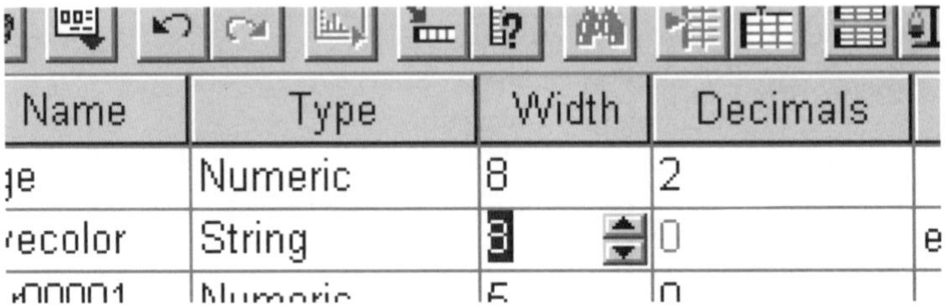

Figure 2.17 Highlighting the default value of the cell in the **Width** column in **Variable View**

4. DECIMALS

This refers to the number of digits to the right of the decimal place for the entries (e.g. enter 2 for **Decimals** in order to input data such as 3.14, etc.). For numeric data, by default this number is usually set to 2. You can alter this in the same way as for the value of the **Width**, as just described and shown in Figures 2.16 and 2.17.

If **Decimals** is not relevant to the data type (e.g. for string data), then **Decimals** is given as a greyed out 0, as shown in Figure 2.11.

5. LABEL

Since the variable name can only be a maximum of eight alphanumeric characters long (see above), you may wish to specify a variable label that is not confined to eight characters. One advantage of doing so is that when you return to **Data View**, if you want quickly to check the meaning of one of your variable names, you can do so simply by placing your cursor over the variable name (at the top of its column) and a few moments later the value label will appear.

Another advantage is that SPSS can display the variable labels in its output windows whenever you carry out statistical tests. This makes it much easier to keep track of what your results mean.

For example, for the data shown in Figure 2.1 (**Data View**), one of the variables is the highest year of school completed. The variable name chosen for this was educ. In the **Variable View** window, this variable is labelled as Highest Year of School Completed. This is shown in Figure 2.2, and more clearly in Figure 2.18, in which this variable is highlighted. (Similarly, for a different dataset, the variable eyecolor is labelled as eye colour in the **Variable View** in Figure 2.11.)

Incidentally, you may have noticed that you cannot read the whole of the highlighted label in Figure 2.18. A quick way of changing the width displayed of a column in either **Variable View** or **Data View** is as follows. Place your cursor on the right-

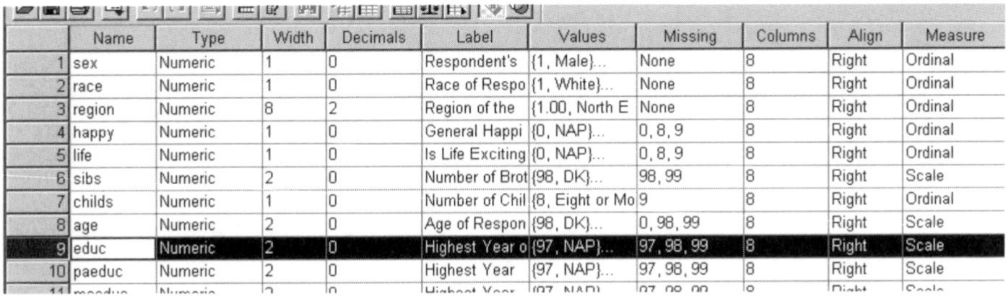

	Name	Type	Width	Decimals	Label	Values	Missing	Columns	Align	Measure
1	sex	Numeric	1	0	Respondent's	{1, Male}...	None	8	Right	Ordinal
2	race	Numeric	1	0	Race of Respo	{1, White}...	None	8	Right	Ordinal
3	region	Numeric	8	2	Region of the	{1.00, North E	None	8	Right	Ordinal
4	happy	Numeric	1	0	General Happi	{0, NAP}...	0, 8, 9	8	Right	Ordinal
5	life	Numeric	1	0	Is Life Exciting	{0, NAP}...	0, 8, 9	8	Right	Ordinal
6	sibs	Numeric	2	0	Number of Brot	{98, DK}...	98, 99	8	Right	Scale
7	childs	Numeric	1	0	Number of Chil	{8, Eight or Mo	9	8	Right	Ordinal
8	age	Numeric	2	0	Age of Respon	{98, DK}...	0, 98, 99	8	Right	Scale
9	educ	Numeric	2	0	Highest Year o	{97, NAP}...	97, 98, 99	8	Right	Scale
10	paeduc	Numeric	2	0	Highest Year	{97, NAP}...	97, 98, 99	8	Right	Scale
11	maaduc	Numeric	2	0	Highest Year	{97, NAP}	97, 98, 99	8	Right	Scale

Figure 2.18 Part of the **Variable View** of Figure 2.2 with the ninth variable, educ, highlighted

hand boundary of the title of the column you wish to re-size, until the cursor changes shape into a vertical black line with both a left and a right arrow. Then drag this cursor to the right (to increase the column width displayed) or the left (to decrease the width displayed) until you are happy.

6. VALUES

Consider the variable eyecolor in the **Variable View** window shown in Figure 2.11. This variable refers to the eye colours of individuals in the dataset. While this is usually a nominal variable (see Chapter 1), if you do not give strings (such as eye colours) numerical values when entering them in **Data View**, you limit the number of statistical operations SPSS can perform on these data. An efficient way of doing this is as follows. Highlight the cell in the sixth column (headed **Values**) of the variable row in **Variable View** (Figure 2.11). You are offered a button with an ellipsis-like symbol (...). Click on this. This brings up the **Value Labels** box, shown in Figure 2.19.

We shall assign the number 1 to the eye colour blue by filling the box as shown in Figure 2.20.

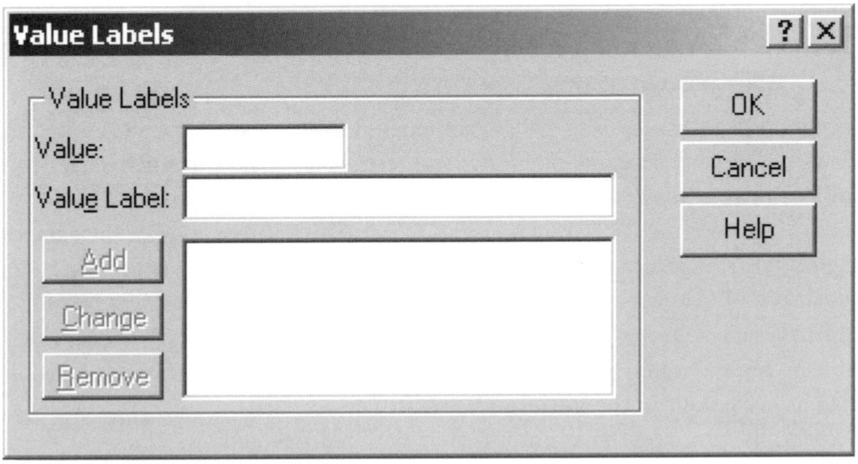

Figure 2.19 The **Value Labels** box

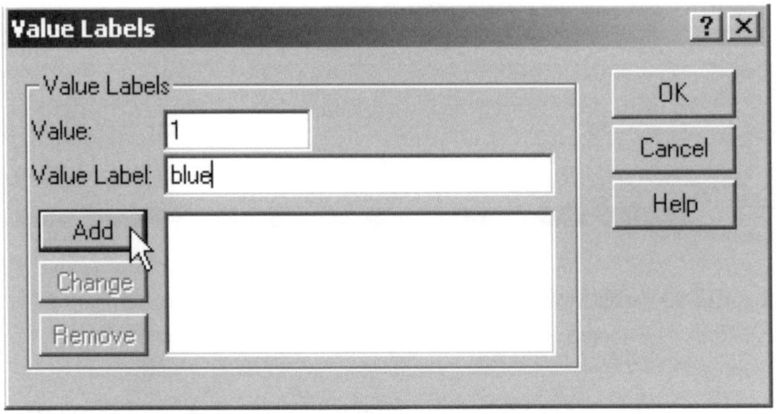

Figure 2.20 Filling in the **Value Labels** box

Then click on the **Add** button, or press the **<Enter>** key on your keyboard. This gives the result shown in Figure 2.21.

Continue adding as many value labels as required (Figure 2.22).

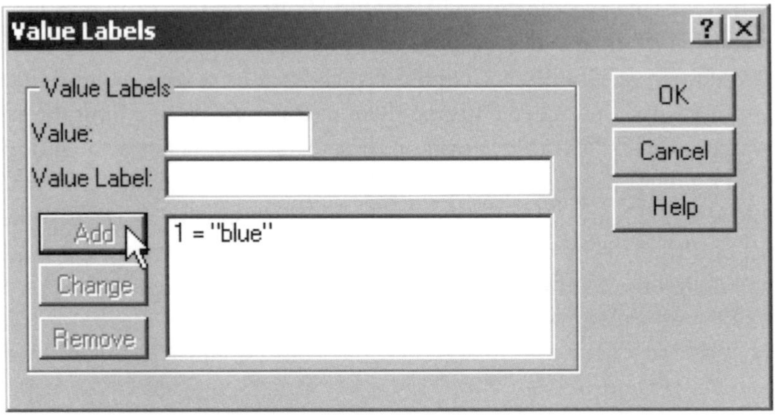

Figure 2.21 The result of clicking on **<Add>**

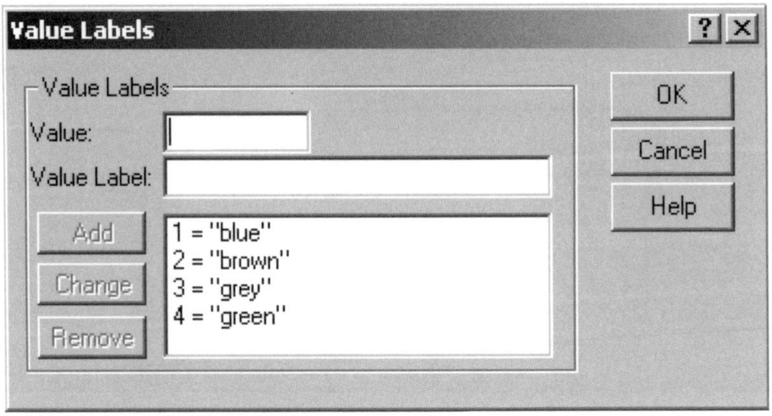

Figure 2.22 A complete list of variable labels

When all the variable labels have been added, click the **OK** button. This closes the **Value Labels** box. If at any time more labels need to be added, or existing ones changed or removed, this can be carried out after re-opening the **Value Labels** box.

In **Data View** you can now enter data in the corresponding variable column. By default, the labels are usually shown, rather than their corresponding numbers (e.g. blue rather than 1, and so on). If this is not your default setting, you can make it so by checking **View\Value Labels** as shown in Figure 2.23.

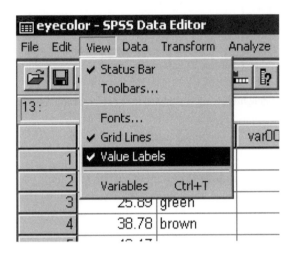

Figure 2.23 Making the display of value labels the default setting

If you do not wish this to be your default setting, but wish to toggle between values (numbers) and labels, you can do so by clicking on the **Value Labels** button on the toolbar, shown in Figure 2.24. (Note that if you cannot remember the function of a button on the toolbar, simply hold the cursor over that button for a moment, and a label will be displayed for it.)

Figure 2.24 The **Value Labels** button on the toolbar

With value labels displayed in **Data View**, simply click (with the left mouse button) on a given cell in the variable column, and this will give you a button in the right-hand side of the cell, as shown in Figure 2.25.

eyecolor – SPSS Data Editor

e Edit View Data Transform Analyze Graphs

eyecolor

	age	eyecolor	var00001
1	19.00	blue	1
2	22.42	brown	0
3	25.89	green	0
4	38.78	brown	1
5	42.17	▼	.
6			

Figure 2.25 The result of highlighting a cell in a column for a non-numerical variable that has value labels in Data View

By clicking on this button, a drop-down menu of the labelled options appears (Figure 2.26), and as soon as you select one of these (by clicking on it) the cell takes its value.

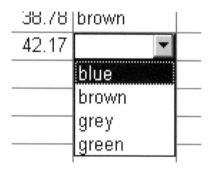

Figure 2.26 Displaying the drop-down menu of labels for a non-numerical variable

7. MISSING

With early versions of SPSS (before the advent of Microsoft Windows) you could not leave any data cells blank and so you would have to specify specific values for missing data; these days you no longer need to do this and so you can leave this blank.

8. COLUMNS

Enter the width of the variable column to be displayed in **Data View**. The default value is usually 8.

9. ALIGN

This allows you to choose the alignment of values displayed in **Data View**. The three options are shown in Figure 2.27.

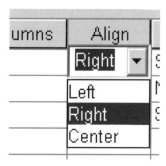

Figure 2.27 The **Data View** alignment options for a variable

10. MEASURE

The final, tenth, column in **View Variable** is where you enter the measurement scale for each variable. Measurement scales were discussed in Chapter 1. The default chosen by SPSS will depend on the data type (specified in 2. Type) for the variable. For example, if the data type is **Date,** then the default measurement scale is scale (see below). The options are accessed from a drop-down menu as shown in Figure 2.28.

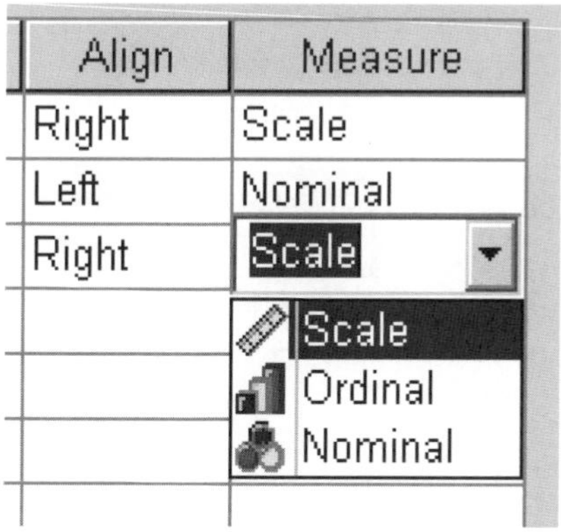

Figure 2.28 The measurement scale options for a variable

These options are:

- Scale – scale data values are numeric on a ratio or interval scale (see Table 1.1)
- Ordinal – ordinal data values are numeric or string values representing distinct categories that have some intrinsic order (see Table 1.1)

- Nominal – nominal data values are numeric or string values representing distinct categories without any intrinsic order (see Table 1.1).

All scale data can be degraded into ordinal data, which in turn can be degraded into nominal data. In general, you should select the highest (scale > ordinal > nominal) measurement scale for which a given variable fulfils the criteria (Table 1.1). Not to do so means that you are deliberately not using the most information available to you, and your statistical tests may be correspondingly less powerful (in a statistical sense).

CONTINGENCY TABLES

So far we have looked at how to enter raw data from actual observations. Sometimes, however, summary data in the form of contingency tables need to be entered. The way to carry this out in SPSS is described in Chapter 7.

SAVING DATA

To save new data that you have entered in **Data View**, select **File\Save**, if you have made changes to a pre-existing data file, or select **File\Save As...** if you are saving a new file or wish to save the changes in a new file (Figure 2.29).

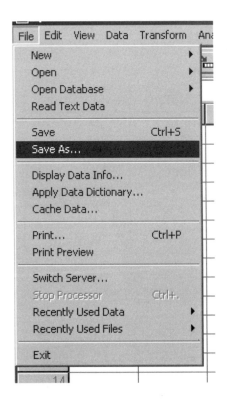

Figure 2.29 Saving data

Alternatively, you can click the **Save** button on the toolbar (Figure 2.30).

Figure 2.30 The **Save** button on the toolbar

Then simply select the appropriate directory (and subdirectory) in which you wish to save your data, and give your data file a suitable name, in the usual way.

OPENING SPSS DATA

To open pre-existing data that have previously been saved in SPSS, you can use **File\Open\Data...**, as shown in Figure 2.31.

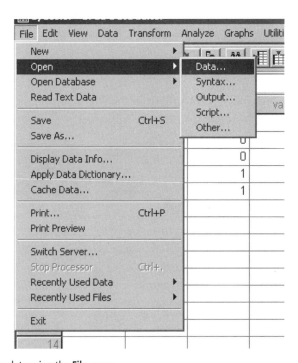

Figure 2.31 Opening data using the **File** menu

Alternatively, you can click the **Open File** button on the toolbar (Figure 2.32).

Figure 2.32 The **Open File** button on the toolbar

This opens the **Open File** box, from which the appropriate data file can be chosen in the usual way (Figure 2.33).

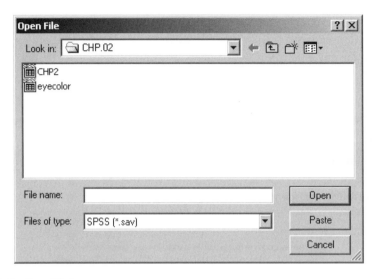

Figure 2.33 The **Open File** box

Recently used data are available directly from the **File** menu: simply (double) click on the data you wish to open (Figure 2.34).

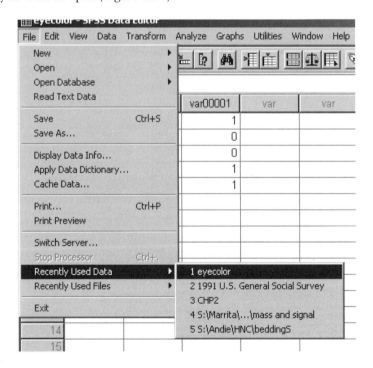

Figure 2.34 Opening recently saved data

READING A SPREADSHEET/DATABASE INTO SPSS

The main difference here from the steps in the last section is that in the **Open File** box you must select the appropriate type of file you require, by clicking on the down arrow with the left mouse button to access the drop-down menu, as shown in Figure 2.35.

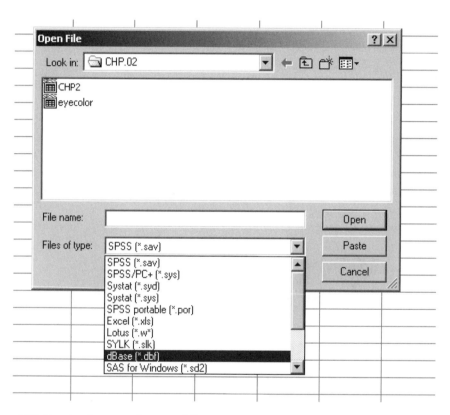

Figure 2.35 Choosing the appropriate type of file

If you have imported a spreadsheet, then its first row will probably contain the variable names, which you must then read into the SPSS data file as follows. Suppose you are opening a Microsoft Excel file. First choose the **Excel (*.xls)** option in the type of file menu shown in Figure 2.35. Then double click on the name of the Excel file you wish to open (or single click on the name and then click **Open**). This will bring up the **Opening File Options** box in which you should check (that is, click in to give the cross symbol) the box labelled **Read Variable Names**, in order that the first row of the spreadsheet is read into variable names (Figure 2.36).

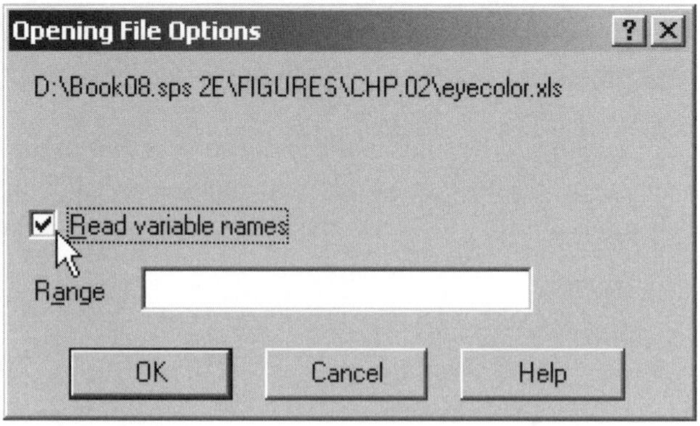

Figure 2.36 Reading column headings of a spreadsheet into SPSS data file variable names

If there are initial empty rows and/or columns in the spreadsheet, then you must also let the SPSS program know the range of cells from which you want to read by entering this in the **Range** box of the **Opening File Options** box. The same format as is used for spreadsheets should be used here. For example, the cells in the rectangle with corners B3 and G10, inclusive, would be entered as B3:G10 (Figure 2.37).

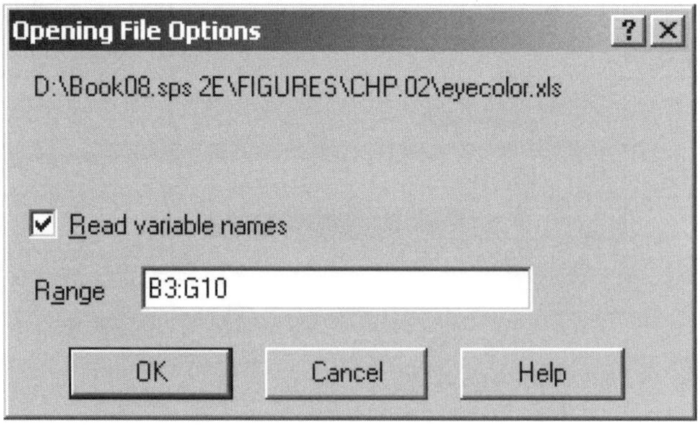

Figure 2.37 Entering the spreadsheet range of cells which are to be read

READING A TEXT DATA FILE INTO SPSS

Suppose you wish to read a text data (ASCII) file such as that shown in Figure 2.38 into SPSS. This file contains two variables, a1 and a2, and the data for these variables are separated by tabs in this case (although they need not be).

```
a1      a2
21      3
22      4
23      45
34      23
35      23
```

Figure 2.38 A sample text data file

First select **File\Read Text Data** from the menu (Figure 2.39).

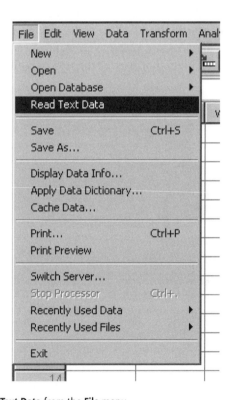

Figure 2.39 Selecting **Read Text Data** from the **File** menu

In the resulting **Open File** box, select the text file you wish to import into SPSS and either double-click it or highlight it and click the **Open** button (Figure 2.40).

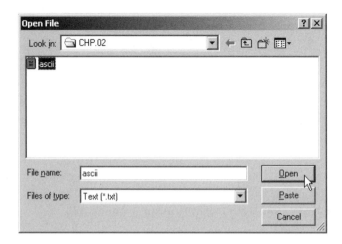

Figure 2.40 The **Open File** box

This causes a Text Import Wizard to be activated. You simply follow each of the six steps as guided. We shall now do this for the text data file shown in Figure 2.38. In the first step, since our text file does not match a predefined format, we choose the **No radio** button (Figure 2.41). Note that part of the text data file is shown in the lower half of the window.

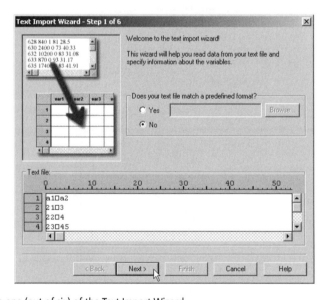

Figure 2.41 Step one (out of six) of the Text Import Wizard

Click on the **Next** button to bring up the window corresponding to the second step. In our case, the data for the two variables are separated by tab spacings (tabs), and so we choose the **Delimited** radio button; we would make the same choice if the separation was by means of another specific character, such as commas. Also, since in this case variable names are included in the first row of our text file, we also choose the radio button labelled **Yes** (Figure 2.42).

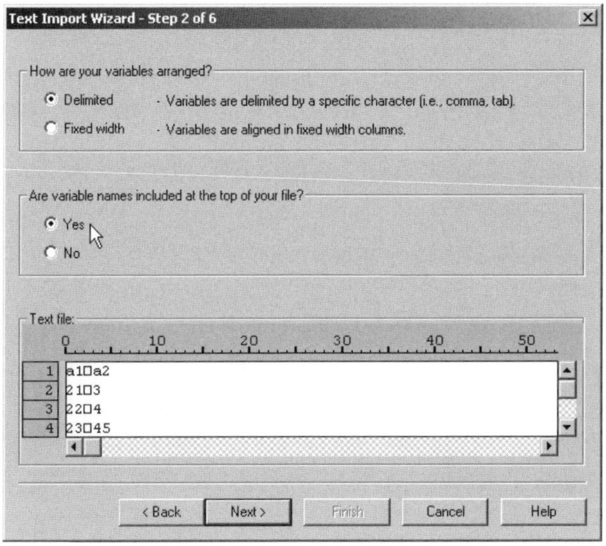

Figure 2.42 Step two (out of six) of the Text Import Wizard

Click on the **Next** button to bring up the window corresponding to the third step. In our case, the first row consists of the variable names, and so the first case of data begins on line number two, and thereafter each line represents a case. Hence we fill in this window as shown in Figure 2.43 (which are the SPSS default settings for this window, since we have already stated that variable names are included in the first row of our text files).

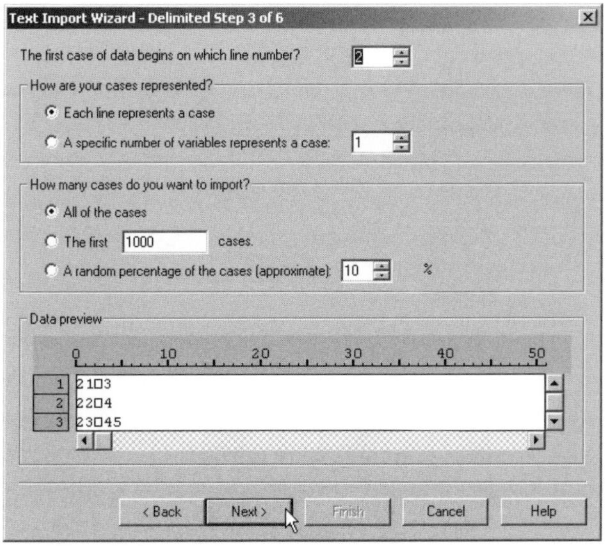

Figure 2.43 Step three (out of six) of the Text Import Wizard

Click on the **Next** button to bring up the window corresponding to the fourth step, in which (in this case) we must state which delimiter is used between variables (Figure 2.44).

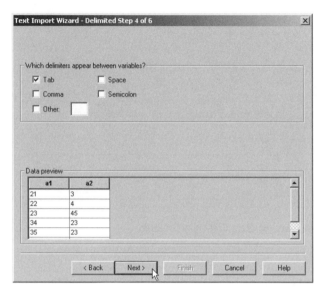

Figure 2.44 Step four (out of six) of the Text Import Wizard

The **Data preview** window shows that our data have been read correctly. Clicking on the **Next** button brings up the window corresponding to the fifth step, in which, in this case, nothing needs to be entered (Figure 2.45).

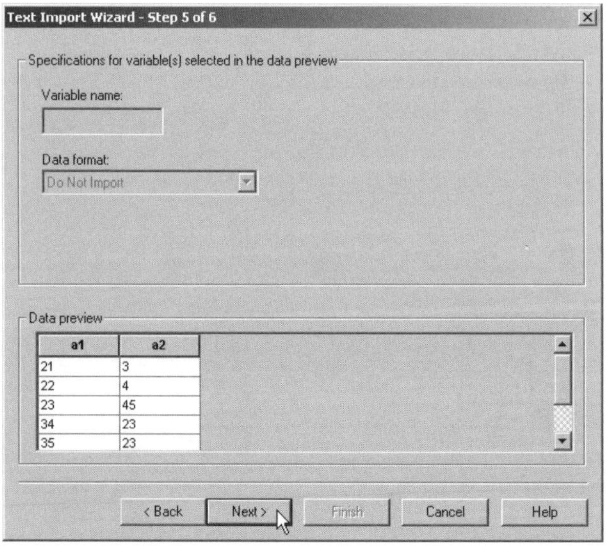

Figure 2.45 Step five (out of six) of the Text Import Wizard

Click on the **Next** button to bring up the window corresponding to the sixth step. This offers you the opportunity to save the file format for future use, which is an option we have not chosen in this case (Figure 2.46).

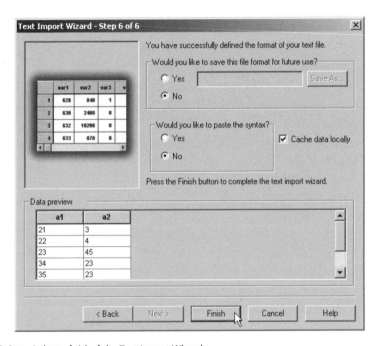

Figure 2.46 Step six (out of six) of the Text Import Wizard

Finally, click on the **Finish** button to bring up the file imported into SPSS (Figure 2.47).

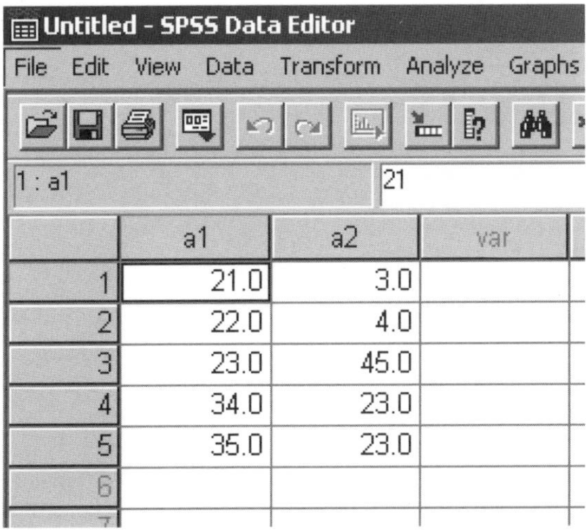

Figure 2.47 The SPSS data corresponding to the sample text data shown in Figure 2.38

chapter 3

CHOOSING A
STATISTICAL TEST

This chapter provides a guide to choosing the right statistical test(s) to run in different circumstances. However, this is not meant to be a replacement for a working knowledge of statistics and the reader is strongly urged to refer to a standard textbook of statistics for further information, including an understanding of why the test(s) chosen is (are) the correct one(s). The choice of appropriate statistical tests should be made before the research project is carried out and the data are collected; in other words, the research should be planned in advance.

Figure 3.1 is a simplified flow diagram showing an overview of some of the choices of statistical tests.

The first decision to make is whether you wish to look for a difference or a correlation between variables.

DIFFERENCES BETWEEN VARIABLES

PARAMETRIC DATA

In this case the data are measured on an interval or ratio scale and fulfil the criteria for parametric tests (see Chapter 1).

If you wish to examine the difference between two such samples that are independent, the independent samples t-test can be used (see Chapter 6). If the two samples are related, the paired samples t-test should be used (see Chapter 6). With more than two samples, an analysis of variance, or ANOVA, should be used (see Chapter 10), as follows.

A one-way ANOVA allows you to test the null hypothesis that the data are a sample from a population in which the mean of a test variable is equal in several independent groups of cases defined by a single grouping variable. The 'one-way' in its name comes from the fact that the cases are allocated to the independent groups on the basis of values for that one test variable. There are no repeated measures.

Simple factorial ANOVA differs from one-way ANOVA in that it can handle several grouping variables (factors) simultaneously. With more than one factor, two types of 'treatment' effects (in ANOVA terminology) can occur: (1) *main effects*, which are the effects of the individual factors; and (2) an *interaction* between factors.

It is useful to run a general factorial ANOVA instead of a simple factorial ANOVA when wishing to control for covariates. (A covariate is a concomitant variable that is measured in addition to the dependent variable in ANOVA, and that represents an

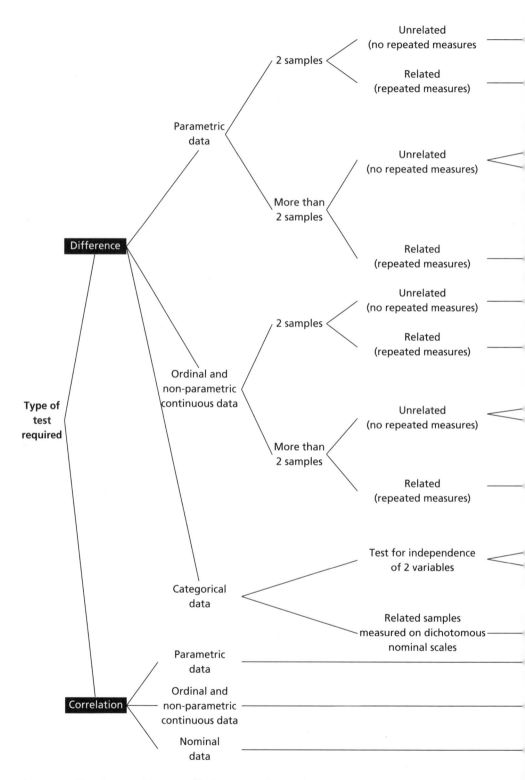

Figure 3.1 A flow diagram giving a simplified overview of some of the choices of statistical tests

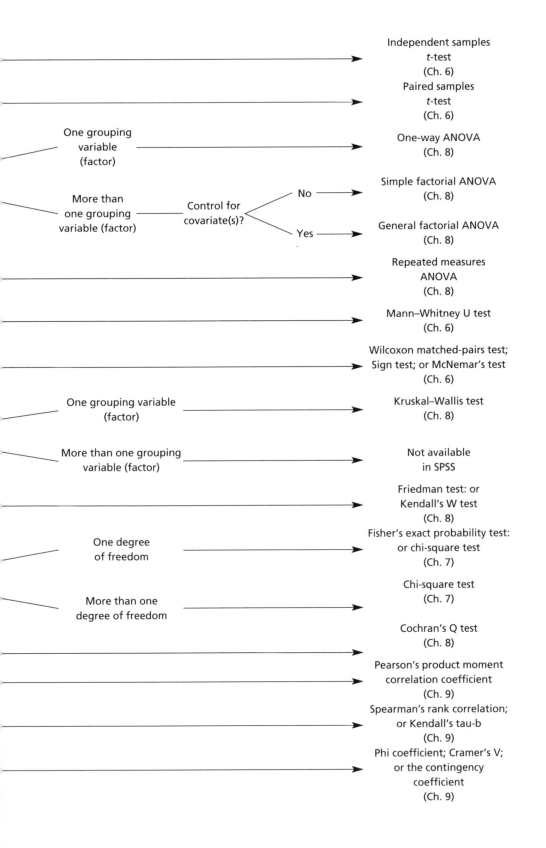

Independent samples
t-test
(Ch. 6)

Paired samples
t-test
(Ch. 6)

One grouping
variable
(factor)

One-way ANOVA
(Ch. 8)

More than
one grouping
variable (factor)

Control for
covariate(s)?

No → Simple factorial ANOVA
(Ch. 8)

Yes → General factorial ANOVA
(Ch. 8)

Repeated measures
ANOVA
(Ch. 8)

Mann–Whitney U test
(Ch. 6)

Wilcoxon matched-pairs test;
Sign test; or McNemar's test
(Ch. 6)

One grouping variable
(factor)

Kruskal–Wallis test
(Ch. 8)

More than one grouping
variable (factor)

Not available
in SPSS

Friedman test: or
Kendall's W test
(Ch. 8)

One degree
of freedom

Fisher's exact probability test:
or chi-square test
(Ch. 7)

More than one
degree of freedom

Chi-square test
(Ch. 7)

Cochran's Q test
(Ch. 8)

Pearson's product moment
correlation coefficient
(Ch. 9)

Spearman's rank correlation;
or Kendall's tau-b
(Ch. 9)

Phi coefficient; Cramer's V;
or the contingency
coefficient
(Ch. 9)

additional, uncontrolled for, source of variation in the dependent variable. For example, in a psychological study of visual perception, age may be a covariate if it has not been controlled for in the experiment.)

A repeated measures ANOVA is used to test hypotheses about the means of a dependent variable when the same dependent variable is measured on more than one occasion for each subject. Between-subjects variables are factors that subdivide the sample into discrete subgroups. Each subject can have only one value for a between-subjects factor. In contrast, within-subjects (repeated measures) variables are factors whose levels are all measured on the same subject. Mixed (split-plot) design experiments have a mixture of these two types of variable.

ORDINAL AND NON-PARAMETRIC CONTINUOUS DATA

If you wish to examine the difference between two such samples that are independent, the Mann–Whitney U test can be used (see Chapter 6). If the two samples are related, SPSS offers the following three choices: the Wilcoxon matched-pairs test; the Sign test; and McNemar's test. Details of these choices are given in Chapter 6.

With more than two samples, a non-parametric ANOVA may be used (see Chapter 8), as follows.

The Kruskal–Wallis test is a non-parametric alternative to the one-way ANOVA and requires that the data be measured at least on an ordinal scale. The test statistic is calculated in the same way as the Mann–Whitney test statistic.

The median test is a non-parametric alternative to the one-way ANOVA that tests whether two or more samples are drawn from populations with the same median. It uses the chi-square statistic.

The Friedman test and Kendall's W test are non-parametric alternatives to the repeated measures ANOVA that are suitable for data measured on at least an ordinal scale.

CATEGORICAL DATA

For categorical data, that is, nominal (qualitative) data or ordinal data assigned to ordered categories, the chi-square test can be carried out to test for independence of two variables (see Chapter 7). For a given contingency table, the chi-square test should not be used if any cell has an expected frequency of less than one or if more than 20% of cells have expected frequencies of less than five. If these criteria are not met and the contingency table has just two rows and two columns, then Fisher's exact probability test can be carried out instead (Chapter 7). If the criteria are not met and there are more than two rows and/or columns, you can try to combine rows and columns so that the criteria are met.

Cochran's Q test is a non-parametric alternative to the repeated measures ANOVA that tests the null hypothesis that the proportion of cases in a particular category is the same for several dichotomous variables (Chapter 10). It is suitable for use when there are related samples measured on dichotomous (binary) nominal scales.

CORRELATION BETWEEN VARIABLES

PARAMETRIC DATA

In this case the data are measured on an interval or ratio scale (see Chapter 1) and fulfil the criteria for parametric tests (see Chapter 1).

If you wish to examine the correlation between two such samples, evaluate Pearson's product moment correlation coefficient (see Chapter 8). A linear regression equation can also be determined (see Chapter 9).

ORDINAL AND NON-PARAMETRIC CONTINUOUS DATA

If you wish to examine the correlation between two such samples, either Spearman's rank correlation or Kendall's tau-b can be evaluated (see Chapter 8).

NOMINAL DATA

SPSS offers the following three measures of association based on the chi-square statistic: the phi coefficient; Cramér's *V*; and the contingency coefficient. These are described in Chapter 9.

chapter 4

EXPLORING DATA AND EDITING GRAPHICAL OUTPUT

A data distribution can be summarized by giving both a measure of its location, for example the mean, and a measure of its dispersion, for example the standard deviation. In addition, it is usually important to have an overview of the shape of the distribution when deciding which statistical tests can be applied.

NOMINAL AND ORDINAL DATA

MEASURES OF CENTRAL TENDENCY

Mode

The mode of a distribution is the value of the observation occurring most frequently. It can be used with all measurement scales.

The highlighted variable in Figure 4.1 is measured on a nominal scale and represents the region of the United States of America in the US General Social Survey data supplied with SPSS (and also shown in Figures 2.1 and 2.2).

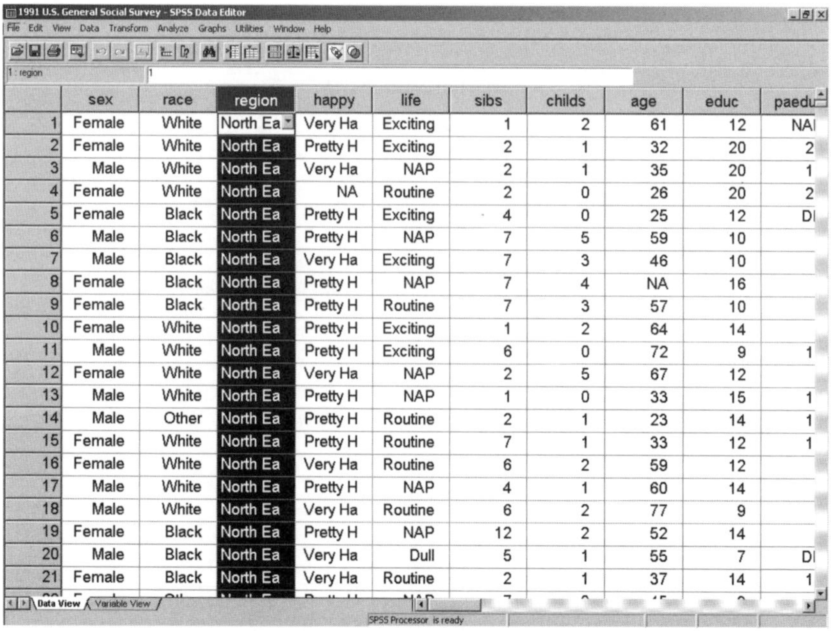

	sex	race	region	happy	life	sibs	childs	age	educ	paedu
1	Female	White	North Ea	Very Ha	Exciting	1	2	61	12	NA
2	Female	White	North Ea	Pretty H	Exciting	2	1	32	20	2
3	Male	White	North Ea	Very Ha	NAP	2	1	35	20	1
4	Female	White	North Ea	NA	Routine	2	0	26	20	2
5	Female	Black	North Ea	Pretty H	Exciting	4	0	25	12	D
6	Male	Black	North Ea	Pretty H	NAP	7	5	59	10	
7	Male	Black	North Ea	Very Ha	Exciting	7	3	46	10	
8	Female	Black	North Ea	Pretty H	NAP	7	4	NA	16	
9	Female	Black	North Ea	Pretty H	Routine	7	3	57	10	
10	Female	White	North Ea	Pretty H	Exciting	1	2	64	14	
11	Male	White	North Ea	Pretty H	Exciting	6	0	72	9	1
12	Female	White	North Ea	Very Ha	NAP	2	5	67	12	
13	Male	White	North Ea	Pretty H	NAP	1	0	33	15	1
14	Male	Other	North Ea	Pretty H	Routine	2	1	23	14	1
15	Female	White	North Ea	Pretty H	Routine	7	1	33	12	1
16	Female	White	North Ea	Very Ha	Routine	6	2	59	12	
17	Male	White	North Ea	Pretty H	NAP	4	1	60	14	
18	Male	White	North Ea	Very Ha	Routine	6	2	77	9	
19	Female	Black	North Ea	Pretty H	NAP	12	2	52	14	
20	Male	Black	North Ea	Very Ha	Dull	5	1	55	7	D
21	Female	Black	North Ea	Very Ha	Routine	2	1	37	14	1

Figure 4.1 Highlighted nominal variable

To determine the mode for this variable, this variable should be recorded as a numeric variable with numerical values corresponding to each of the categories (see Chapter 2). Using **Analyze\Descriptive Statistics\Frequencies...** open the **Frequencies** box (as shown in Figure 4.2).

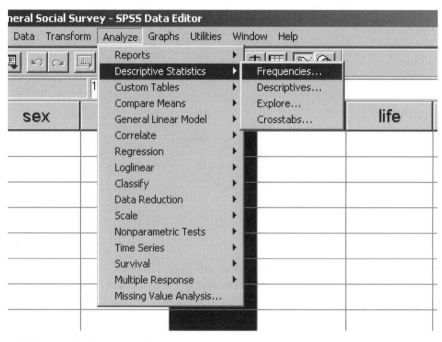

Figure 4.2 Opening the **Frequencies** box

In the **Frequencies** box select the required variable (region) and move it into the **Variable(s)** section by clicking the arrow button (Figure 4.3).

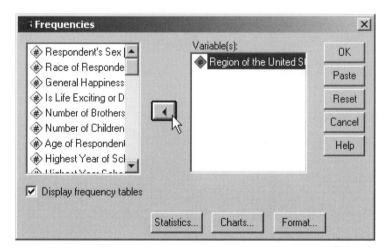

Figure 4.3 The **Frequencies** box

Click on the **Statistics...** button to open the **Frequencies: Statistics** box. Select **Mode** under **Central Tendency** (Figure 4.4) and then click **Continue**.

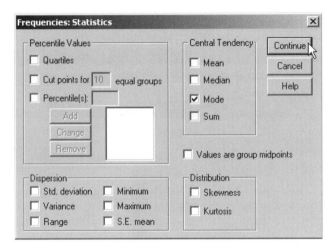

Figure 4.4 The **Frequencies: Statistics** box

On returning to the **Frequencies** box, click **OK**. This takes you to the **Output** screen where the value label corresponding to the mode is stated (in this case 1.00 = North East), as required (Figure 4.5), together with the number of valid and missing cases. The frequency table for the variable appears underneath the box containing the mode, as we left **Display frequency tables** checked (the default mode) in the **Frequencies** box (see Figure 4.3).

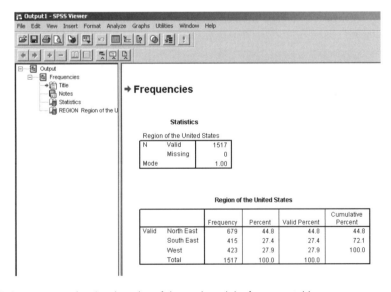

Figure 4.5 Output screen showing the value of the mode and the frequency table

Median

The median is the middle value of a set of observations ranked in order and can be used with measurement scales that are at least ordinal (that is, ordinal, interval or ratio).

Staying with the US General Social Survey data, we can consider the variable occcat80, which represents occupational category (highlighted variable in Figure 4.6) to be ordinal.

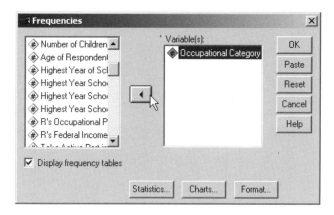

	sibs	childs	age	educ	paeduc	maeduc	speduc	prestg80	occcat80	tax
1	1	2	61	12	NAP	12	NAP	22	Service	Too Hig
2	2	1	32	20	20	18	20	75	Manageri	Too Hig
3	2	1	35	20	16	14	17	59	Manageri	NA
4	2	0	26	20	20	20	NAP	48	Manageri	Too Hig
5	4	0	25	12	DK	DK	NAP	42	Service	Too Hig
6	7	5	59	10	8	6	NAP	DK,NA,N	.	NA
7	7	3	46	10	8	DK	NAP	DK,NA,N	.	DI
8	7	4	NA	16	5	6	NAP	60	Technical	NA
9	7	3	57	10	6	5	NAP	DK,NA,N	.	DI
10	1	2	64	14	8	12	20	38	Operation	Too Hig
11	6	0	72	9	12	DK	NAP	36	Operation	Too Hig
12	2	5	67	12	8	8	13	28	Operation	NA
13	1	0	33	15	11	12	14	65	Manageri	NA
14	2	1	23	14	12	12	NAP	49	Technical	Too Hig
15	7	1	33	12	12	12	NAP	50	Technical	Too Hig
16	6	2	59	12	8	DK	12	DK,NA,N	.	Too Hig
17	4	1	60	14	6	6	NAP	32	Technical	NA
18	6	2	77	9	0	0	8	36	Operation	About Ri
19	12	2	52	14	8	12	8	51	Technical	NA
20	5	1	55	7	DK	DK	16	42	Service	Too Hig
21	2	1	37	14	12	12	NAP	42	Service	Too Hig
22	7	0	45	9	8	NA	NAP	DK,NA,N	.	NA
23	4	0	34	12	DK	DK	DK	42	Service	DI
24	7	3	35	9	DK	DK	9	DK,NA,N	.	DI

Figure 4.6 Highlighted ordinal variable

To determine the median for this variable, this variable should be recorded as a numeric variable with numerical values corresponding to each of the categories (see Chapter 2). Open the **Frequencies** box as shown above in Figure 4.2. In the **Frequencies** box select the required variable and move it into the **Variable(s)** section by clicking the arrow button (Figure 4.7).

Figure 4.7 The **Frequencies** box

Click on the **Statistics** button to open the **Frequencies: Statistics box**. Select Median under **Central Tendency** (Figure 4.8) and then click **Continue**.

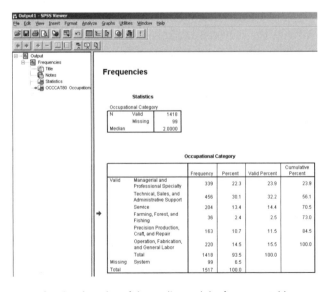

Figure 4.8 The **Frequencies: Statistics** box

On returning to the **Frequencies** box, click **OK**. This takes you to the **Output** screen where the value label corresponding to the median is stated (in this case 2.0000 = Technical, Sales, and Administrative Support), as required (Figure 4.9), together with the number of valid and missing cases. Again, the frequency table for the variable appears underneath the box containing the median, as we left **Display frequency tables** checked (the default mode) in the **Frequencies** box (see Figure 4.7).

Frequencies

Statistics

Occupational Category

N	Valid	1418
	Missing	99
Median		2.0000

Occupational Category

		Frequency	Percent	Valid Percent	Cumulative Percent
Valid	Managerial and Professional Specialty	339	22.3	23.9	23.9
	Technical, Sales, and Administrative Support	456	30.1	32.2	56.1
	Service	204	13.4	14.4	70.5
	Farming, Forest, and Fishing	36	2.4	2.5	73.0
	Precision Production, Craft, and Repair	163	10.7	11.5	84.5
	Operation, Fabrication, and General Labor	220	14.5	15.5	100.0
	Total	1418	93.5	100.0	
Missing	System	99	6.5		
Total		1517	100.0		

Figure 4.9 Output screen showing the value of the median and the frequency table

DISTRIBUTION SHAPE

Diagrammatic representation
Nominal and ordinal data can be represented by bar charts and pie charts.

Bar chart

Suppose we wish to represent the nominal variable highlighted in Figure 4.1 as a bar chart. First open the **Frequencies** box (Figure 4.2) and select the required variable (Figure 4.3). Then click on the **Charts...** button, to open the **Frequencies: Charts** box. Choose the **Bar chart(s)** radio button and decide whether you would like the axis label display to be in frequencies or percentages (Figure 4.10).

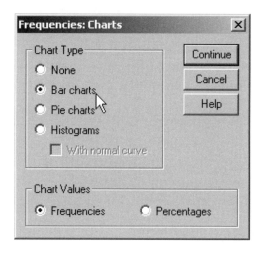

Figure 4.10 The **Frequencies: Charts** box

Click on **Continue** and then, in the **Frequencies** box, click on **OK**. This takes you to the **Output** window, where the bar chart has been created (Figure 4.11).

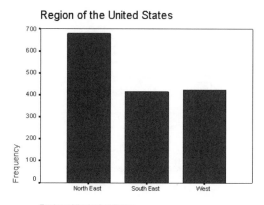

Figure 4.11 Bar chart

The bar chart, and indeed all graphical output, can be readily edited in SPSS as described below.

An alternative way of obtaining a bar chart is using **Graphs\Bar...** in **Data View** (Figure 4.12).

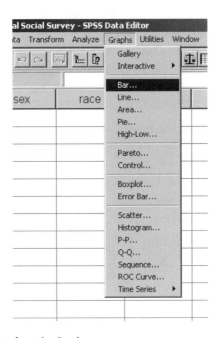

Figure 4.12 Selecting bar charts from the **Graphs** menu

This opens the **Bar Charts** box (Figure 4.13).

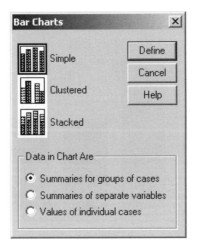

Figure 4.13 The **Bar Charts** box

Select the type of chart you want and then click **Define** to take you to the **Define Simple Bar** box, in which you make the appropriate choices (see Figure 4.14) and then click **OK** to obtain the bar chart as before. (If you wish to give your bar chart a title and subtitle at this stage, simply click on the **Titles...** button in the **Define Simple Bar** box first and fill in the next box appropriately.)

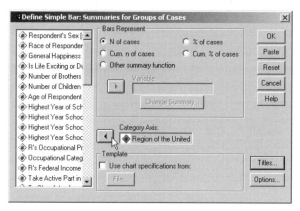

Figure 4.14 The **Define Simple Bar** box

Note that in the bar chart produced by SPSS, categories for which the frequency is zero do not appear.

Pie chart
Nominal and ordinal data can also be represented by pie charts (pie diagrams). As for bar charts, there are two methods of creating a pie chart. These will be illustrated for the nominal variable which appears in Figure 4.1 (regions of the United States of America). The first method is to begin by opening the **Frequencies** box by selecting **Analyze\Descriptive Statistics\Frequencies...** (Figure 4.2) and selecting the required variable (Figure 4.3). Then click on the **Charts...** button to open the **Frequencies: Charts** box. Choose the **Pie chart(s)** radio button and decide whether you would like the chart values displayed to be frequencies or percentages (Figure 4.15).

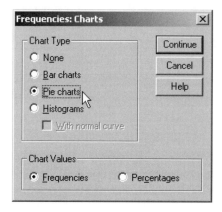

Figure 4.15 The **Frequencies: Charts** box

The second method is to select **Graphs\Pie...** in **Data View** (Figure 4.16).

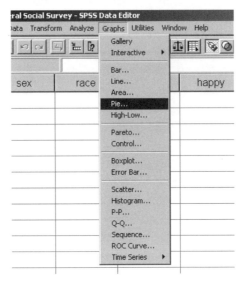

Figure 4.16 Selecting pie charts from the **Graphs** menu

This leads to the **Pie Charts** box, in which, after selecting the appropriate radio button (Figure 4.17), you should click on **Define**.

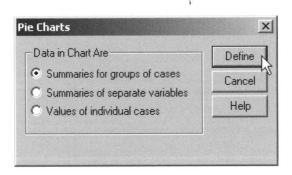

Figure 4.17 The **Pie Charts** box

This opens the **Define Pie** box, in which you make the appropriate choices (see Figure 4.18); in this case we have opted for the slices to represent percentages (that is, the number in each category is expressed as a percentage of the total number).

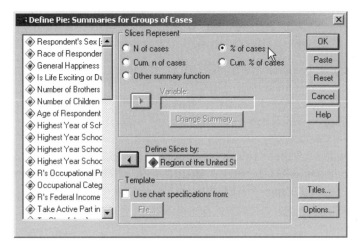

Figure 4.18 The **Define Pie** box

Clicking **OK** in either the **Frequencies: Charts** box (Figure 4.15: the first method) or in the **Define Pie** box (Figure 4.18: the second method) then takes you to the **Output** window and the required pie chart (Figure 4.19).

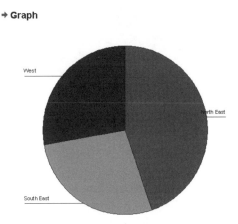

Figure 4.19 Pie chart

The next subsection describes how to edit this pie chart, for example in order to display the percentages.

Editing graphical outputs
In order to move into the edit mode for any graphical output, just double-click on the graph in **Output**. This will take you into the Chart Editor. Here, you can edit many aspects, such as the:

1. Title and subtitle
2. Labelling

3. Fonts
4. Colour scheme
5. Fill pattern
6. Categories (one or more can be deleted)
7. Axes (which can be swapped)
8. Chart type (for example from a bar chart into a pie chart, and *vice versa*)
9. Scale axis range (which can be changed).

To illustrate a few of these editing capabilities, we will edit the pie and bar charts produced above (shown in Figures 4.19 and 4.11, respectively). On double-clicking the pie chart, you enter the Chart Editor, as shown in Figure 4.20.

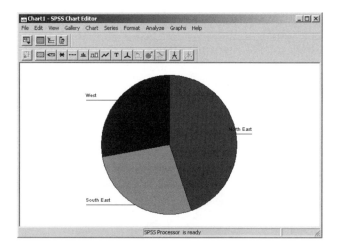

Figure 4.20 Chart Editor

Once in the Chart Editor, you often have three options for editing features:

- From the menus
- By using the toolbar
- By double-clicking the feature to be edited.

Pick whichever of these options you prefer. The option of double-clicking individual features is often the easiest to use, and will mainly be used here.

1. Title and subtitle
In the case of the pie chart in Figure 4.20 we do not have a pre-existing title on which to double-click. So we select **Chart\Title...** from the menu, as shown in Figure 4.21.

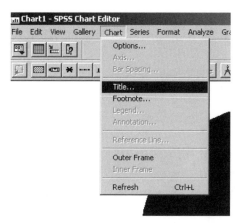

Figure 4.21 Selecting title from the **Chart** menu

This opens the **Titles** box, which you can fill in with a suitable title and subtitle (if required), and edit the justification of these (centre by default) (Figure 4.22).

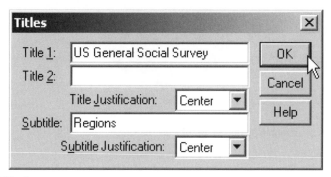

Figure 4.22 The **Titles** box

Clicking **<OK>** then gives the corresponding changes to the chart, as shown in Figure 4.23.

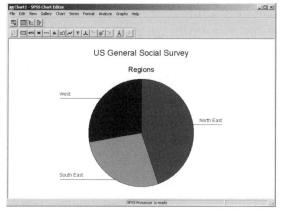

Figure 4.23 Edited pie chart with title and subtitle

2. *Labelling*

Suppose we now wish to show the percentages in the labels of the pie chart of Figure 4.23. If you simply double-click on any of the labels, each existing label becomes surrounded by four small black editing squares and the **Pie Options** box opens. This is shown in Figure 4.24.

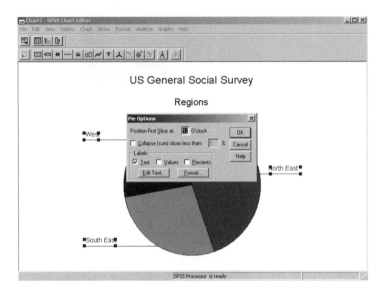

Figure 4.24 The result of double-clicking a label of a pie chart

There are several options available in the **Pie Options** box:

- **Position First Slice at** – this allows you to change the positions of the slices (by altering the position of the first slice)
- **Collapse (sum) slices less than _ %** – this allows you to combine all slices less than a percentage that you specify
- **Labels** – this allows you to display any combination of text, values and percentages as labels
- **Edit Text...** – this allows you to edit the text used to label the slices, and to give a name to a collapsed slice (other than 'other')
- **Format...** – this allows you to edit the position and format of the labels.

We will just add percentages to the labels. We do this by checking **Percents**, as shown in Figure 4.25.

Clicking **<OK>** then gives the corresponding changes to the chart, as shown in Figure 4.26. (Just click anywhere inside the Chart Editor but away from the pie chart to get rid of the four small black editing squares surrounding each label.)

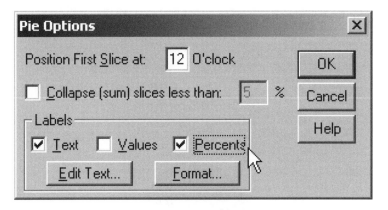

Figure 4.25 The **Pie Options** box

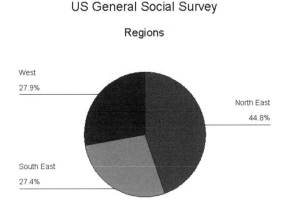

Figure 4.26 Pie chart with percentages

3. Fonts

Suppose we now wish to change the font used for the main title in Figure 4.26. We click once on the main title and then click the **Text** button, shown in Figure 4.27.

Figure 4.27 The **Text** button

This opens the **Text Styles** box, as shown in Figure 4.28.

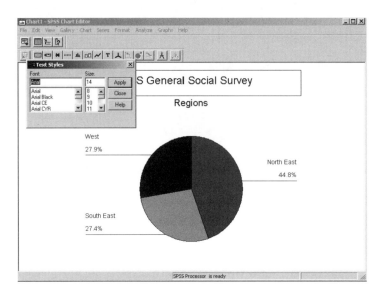

Figure 4.28 Opening the **Text Styles** box

We choose **Times New Roman** (from the scrollable menu) for the chart title, in font size 14, and then click **<Apply>**. This changes the title font, as shown in Figure 4.29.

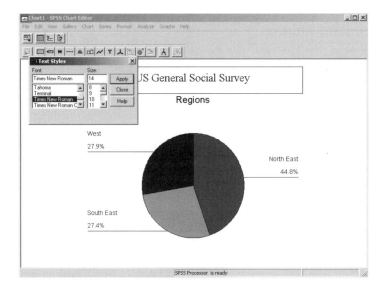

Figure 4.29 Changing the title font

Suppose we now wish to change the subtitle font to Times New Roman and size 11. We simply click on the subtitle, whereupon the details given in the **Text Styles** box now change to those of the subtitle, and then we make the changes shown in Figure 4.30.

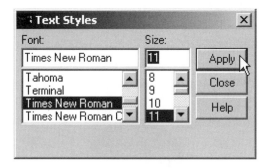

Figure 4.30 The **Text Styles** box

Click on **<Apply>** to implement the change. If there are no further font changes you wish to make, then click **<Close>**. (To deselect the subtitle, simply click anywhere in the Chart Editor once.) The result is shown in Figure 4.31.

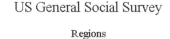

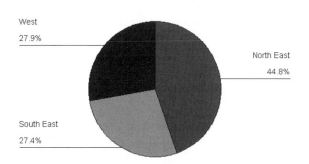

Figure 4.31 The Pie chart with a font change to the title and subtitle

You can edit the fonts of the slice labels and of the percentages in the same way.

4. *Colour scheme*
In Chart Editor you can use the **Color** button to change colours (Figure 4.32).

Figure 4.32 The **Color** button

For example, if you wish to change the colour of any sectors of the pie chart of Figure 4.31, just click once in each appropriate sector and then click the **Color** button. This opens the **Colors** box; Figure 4.33 shows the result.

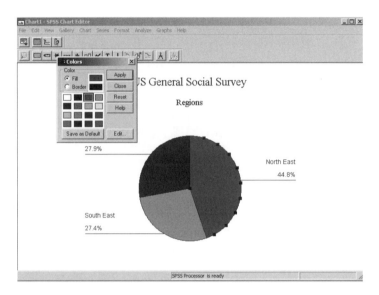

Figure 4.33 Editing a pie chart sector colour

Suppose you want to change the colour of the sector chosen in Figure 4.33 to white, and to keep a black boundary. The appropriate changes to make in the **Colors** box are shown in Figure 4.34.

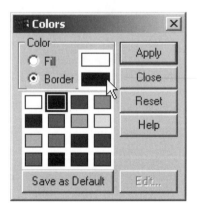

Figure 4.34 The **Colors** box

After clicking **<Apply>** and **<Close>** the edited pie chart has the appearance shown in Figure 4.35.

US General Social Survey

Regions

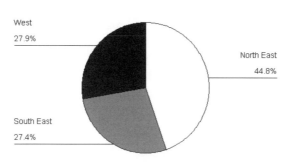

Figure 4.35 The Pie chart after editing the colour of one of its sectors

5. Fill Pattern

It is often useful to change the type of shading used in the graphical output of SPSS. For example, you may wish to print in monochrome rather than in colour. Different sectors of a pie chart, for instance, can usefully be given different fill patterns to differentiate the sectors more readily. We shall do this for the pie chart in Figure 4.35. The **Fill Pattern** button is just to the left of the **Color** button, as shown in Figure 4.36.

Figure 4.36 The Fill Pattern button

Select a sector of the pie chart and click on it. Then click on the **Fill Pattern** button. This opens the **Fill Patterns** box, as shown in Figure 4.37.

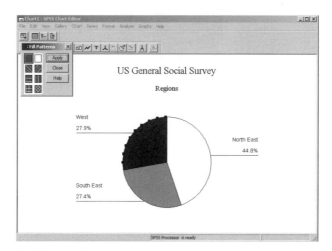

Figure 4.37 Opening the Fill Patterns box

Make your choice of pattern and then click **<Apply>**, as shown in Figure 4.38.

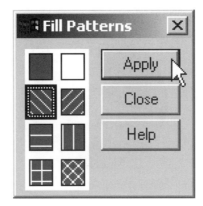

Figure 4.38 The **Fill Patterns** box

You can also change the fill pattern of the other non-white sector if you wish, in the same way. After doing this and then clicking **<Close>**, the resulting pie chart is as shown in Figure 4.39.

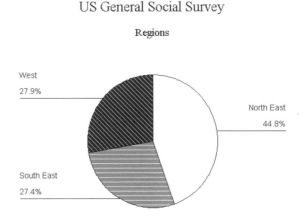

Figure 4.39 The Pie chart after editing the fill pattern of two of its sectors

6. Categories

Consider again the bar chart shown in Figure 4.11. Suppose we wished to remove the category South East. Double-click on a bar in Chart Editor. This opens the **Bar/Line/Area Displayed Data** box. This is shown in Figure 4.40, in which the colour scheme for the bars has also been changed to make it easier to follow in the monochromatic printouts available in this book.

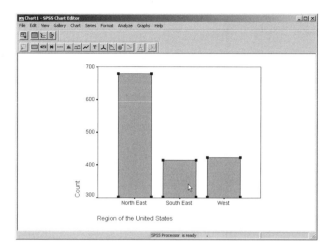

Figure 4.40 Opening the **Bar/Line/Area Displayed Data** box

In the **Bar/Line/Area Displayed Data** box, move the selected category (South East) from the **Display** list to the **Omit** list. This is shown in Figure 4.41.

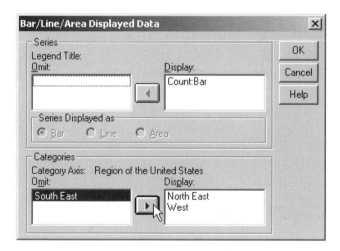

Figure 4.41 The **Bar/Line/Area Displayed Data** box

After clicking **<OK>** the resulting edited bar chart has the appearance shown in Figure 4.42.

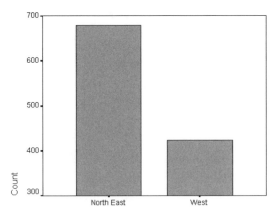

Figure 4.42 The Bar chart after removing one of its categories

7. *Axes*

Two axes can be swapped around in a graph. This is achieved in Chart Editor by clicking the **Swap Axes** button (Figure 4.43).

Figure 4.43 The **Swap Axes** button

The result of clicking the **Swap Axes** button on the bar chart of Figure 4.42 is shown in Figure 4.44.

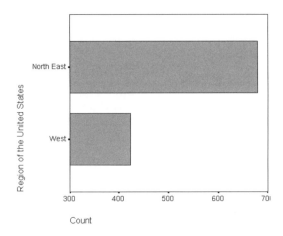

Figure 4.44 The bar chart after swapping its axes

8. *Chart type*

You can readily change between different graphical representations in Chart Editor by selecting the appropriate option available from **Gallery** in the menu. Suppose, for instance, that you were starting with the pie chart shown in Figure 4.19. Selecting **Gallery** when you have a pie chart or bar chart in Chart Editor gives you the options shown in Figure 4.45.

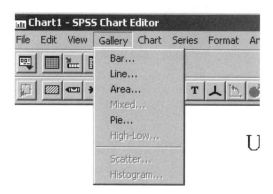

Figure 4.45 The **Gallery** menu

To change the pie chart into the corresponding bar chart, simply select **Gallery\Bar...**, which opens the **Bar Charts** box. This is shown in Figure 4.46.

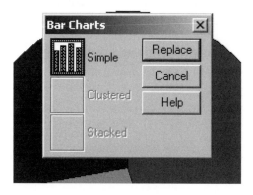

Figure 4.46 Opening the **Bar Charts** box from the **Gallery** menu

In this case you can see that only one type of bar chart is offered, corresponding to the type of pie chart data currently represented in the Chart Editor. Clicking on **<Replace>** in the **Bar Charts** box immediately closes the **Bar Charts** box and replaces the pie chart with a bar chart. This is shown in Figure 4.47. Note that any editing of colours and fill patterns you may have carried out on the first chart (the pie chart in this case) is not carried over into the second chart (the bar chart in this case). Such

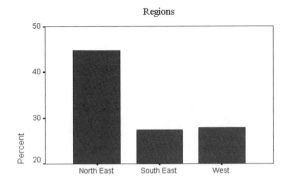

Figure 4.47 The result of swapping a pie chart into a bar chart

editing is permanently lost, in the sense that swapping back again (in this case from bar chart to pie chart) does not recover your colour and fill pattern editing.

Finishing editing

The ninth form of editing mentioned above, namely of the scale axis range, is described in the next major section of this chapter, which deals with interval and ratio (scale) data.

When you have finished editing a chart in Chart Editor, close Chart Editor to return to the SPSS Output window, which will now contain the edited version of your chart. You may close Chart Editor by selecting **File\Close** from the menu (Figure 4.48), or by clicking on the **Close** button which, as in most Windows programs, is found in the top right-hand corner (Figure 4.49).

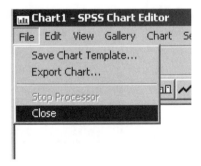

Figure 4.48 Selecting **Close** from the **File** menu

Figure 4.49 The **Close** button

Frequencies

As seen above, tables of frequencies may be obtained by using **Analyze\Descriptive Statistics\Frequencies…** to open the **Frequencies** box (as shown in Figure 4.2). Remember to leave **Display frequency tables** checked (the default mode) in the **Frequencies** box (see Figure 4.3).

INTERVAL AND RATIO DATA

MEASURES OF CENTRAL TENDENCY

Mode and median

See above.

Arithmetic mean

The (arithmetic) mean ($\bar{x}$) is the average value of a distribution (the sum of all the values divided by the number of cases; Equation 4.1) and can be used for continuous data, that is, data measured on an interval or ratio scale.

$$\bar{x} = \frac{1}{n} \sum_{i=1}^{n} x_i \qquad (4.1)$$

The highlighted variable (age) in Figure 4.50 is measured on a ratio scale and represents the age in years of respondents in the 1991 US General Social Survey data supplied with SPSS.

sibs	childs	age	educ	pa
1	2	61 ▾	12	
2	1	32	20	
2	1	35	20	
2	0	26	20	
4	0	25	12	
7	5	59	10	
7	3	46	10	
7	4	NA	16	
7	3	57	10	
1	2	64	14	
6	0	72	9	
2	5	67	12	
1	0	33	15	
2	1	23	14	
7	1	33	12	
6	2	59	12	
4	1	60	14	

Figure 4.50 Highlighted continuous (ratio) variable

One method of obtaining the mean of this variable is to select **Descriptive Statistics\Descriptives...** as shown in Figure 4.51.

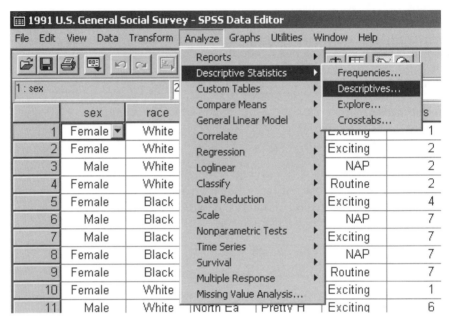

Figure 4.51 Selecting **Descriptives...** from the **Descriptive Statistics** menu

Select the required variable (whose mean you wish to obtain) as shown in Figure 4.52.

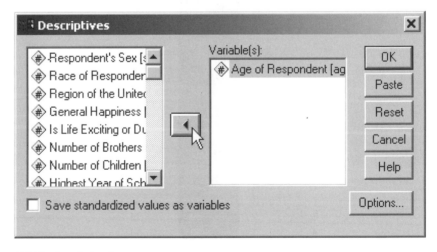

Figure 4.52 The **Descriptives** box

Then click **OK**. By default, the corresponding **Output** (shown in Figure 4.53) will contain the minimum and maximum values, the mean and the standard deviation. From this it can be seen that the mean age is 45.63 years.

Descriptive Statistics

	N	Minimum	Maximum	Mean	Std. Deviation
Age of Respondent	1514	18	89	45.63	17.808
Valid N (listwise)	1514				

Figure 4.53 **Output** screen showing the default values obtained from **Descriptives**

(Alternatively, you can also use **Analyze\Descriptive Statistics\Frequencies...** to open the **Frequencies** box (shown in Figure 4.2). In the **Frequencies** box select the required variable and move it into the **Variable(s)** section by clicking the arrow button (Figure 4.3). Deselect **Display frequency tables**. Click on the **Statistics...** button to open the **Frequencies: Statistics** box. Select **Mean** under **Central Tendency** and then click **Continue**. On returning to the **Frequencies** box, click **OK**. This takes you to the **Output** screen where the required mean (45.63 years) appears.

MEASURES OF DISPERSION

Range

The range is the difference between the smallest and largest values in a distribution and can be used for data measured on an interval or ratio scale.

The range can be obtained by carrying out the same procedure as for the mean (see above), but this time in the **Descriptives** box (Figure 4.52) click on **Options...** to open the **Descriptives: Options** box. Simply check **Range** in the **Descriptives: Options** box, as shown in Figure 4.54.

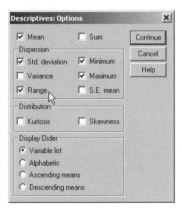

Figure 4.54 The **Descriptives: Options** box – obtaining the range

Click on **Continue** to return to the **Descriptives** box, and then on **OK**. The resulting Output for the age of respondents in the 1991 US General Social Survey is shown in Figure 4.55, from which it can be seen that the range is 71 years (with the minimum age being 18 years, and the maximum 89 years).

Descriptive Statistics

	N	Range	Minimum	Maximum	Mean	Std. Deviation
Age of Respondent	1514	71	18	89	45.63	17.808
Valid N (listwise)	1514					

Figure 4.55 Output screen showing the value of the range

Measures relating to quantiles

Quartiles divide the ordered data into four equal groups, so that each group contains a quarter of the observations. Thus a quarter (25%) of the observations lie below the first quartile, and a further quarter (25%) of the observations lie between the first and second quartiles. Since half (50%) of the observations lie below (and above) the second quartile, this means that the second quartile is also the median (see above). The interquartile range is the difference between the third and the first quartile, and contains 50% of the observations.

To obtain the quartiles for the age of respondents in the US General Social Survey (Figure 4.50) first carry out the same procedure as for the mean (see above) to obtain the **Frequencies: Statistics** box. Select **Quartiles** (Figure 4.56). (If you wish to obtain other percentiles, use the other boxes in the **Percentile Values** section accordingly. For example, in order to obtain deciles, check **Cut points** for 10 equal groups.)

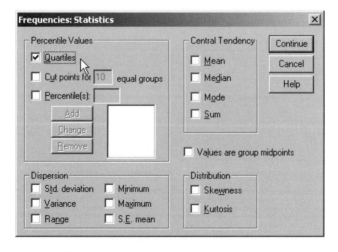

Figure 4.56 The **Frequencies: Statistics** box – obtaining quartiles

Click on **Continue** to return to the **Frequencies** box and then on **OK**. The resulting **Output** is shown in Figure 4.57, in which the values of the first quartile (25 Percentile), median or second quartile (50 Percentile) and third quartile (75 Percentile) are given as 32, 41 and 60 years, respectively. The interquartile range is obtained by subtracting the value of the first quartile from that of the third quartile, and in this case is $60 - 32 = 28$ years.

Statistics

Age of Respondent

N	Valid	1514
	Missing	3
Percentiles	25	32.00
	50	41.00
	75	60.00

Figure 4.57 Output screen showing the values of the quartiles

The semi-interquartile range or quartile deviation is one-half of the difference between the third and the first quartile. It is calculated by subtracting the value of the first quartile from that of the third quartile, as above, and then dividing the result by two. In the case of the age of respondents in the US General Social Survey (Figure 4.50) the semi-interquartile range or quartile deviation = 28/2 = 14 years.

The 10 to 90 percentile range, or interdecile range, is the difference between the 90th and 10th (per)centiles, or equivalently, between the ninth and first deciles.

To obtain the 10 to 90 percentile (interdecile) range for the age of respondents in the US General Social Survey (Figure 4.50) first carry out the same procedure as for the mean (see above) to obtain the **Frequencies: Statistics** box. Select **Percentiles** and **type 10** in the box to the right of it, as shown in Figure 4.58. Click on **Add**. This selects the 10th percentile.

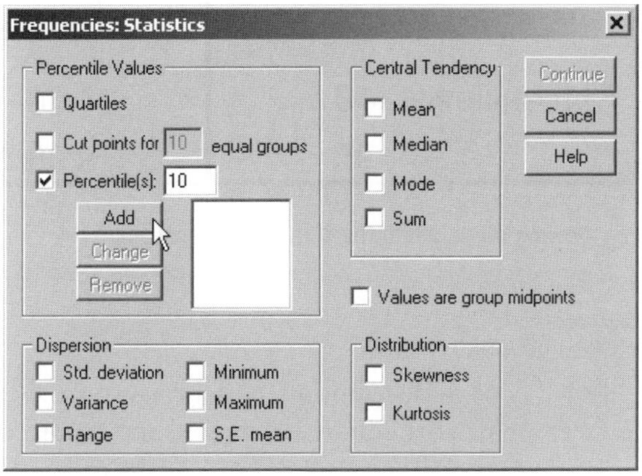

Figure 4.58 The **Frequencies: Statistics** box – obtaining the 10th percentile

To obtain the 90th percentile, repeat the process with 90 this time. After clicking on **Add**, the **Frequencies: Statistics** box should appear as in Figure 4.59.

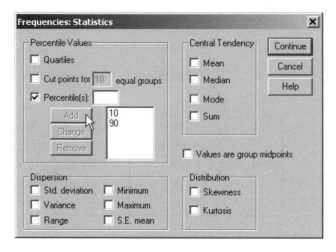

Figure 4.59 The **Frequencies: Statistics** box – obtaining the 10th and 90th percentiles

Click on **Continue** to return to the **Frequencies** box and then on **OK**. The resulting Output is shown in Figure 4.60, in which the values of the 10th and 90th percentiles are respectively given as 24 and 73 years. The 10 to 90 percentile (interdecile) range is obtained by subtracting the value of the 10th percentile from the 90th percentile, and in this case is equal to 73 – 24 = 49 years.

Statistics

Age of Respondent

N	Valid	1514
	Missing	3
Percentiles	10	24.00
	90	73.00

Figure 4.60 Output screen showing the values of the 10th and 90th percentiles

Standard deviation

The standard deviation (s) of a distribution is a measure of dispersion based on deviations from the mean (which are squared, summed and (approximately) averaged and then the square root is taken), has the same units as the original observations, and can be used for data measured on an interval or ratio scale. To calculate the standard deviation, the sum of the squared deviations from the mean is divided by $(n - 1)$, where n is the number of observations, and then the square root of the result is taken:

$$s = \sqrt{\frac{\sum_{i=1}^{n} (x_i - \bar{x})^2}{n - 1}} \qquad (4.2)$$

The standard deviation can be obtained by carrying out the same procedure as described above for obtaining the mean, by selecting **Descriptive Statistics\Descriptives...** (Figures 4.51 and 4.52). For example, from the Output shown in Figure 4.53, it can be seen that the standard deviation for the age of respondents in the US General Social Survey (Figure 4.50) is approximately 17.8 years.

(An alternative method is to use the **Analyze\Descriptive Statistics\Frequencies...** menu as described above.)

Variance

The variance (s^2) is the square of the standard deviation, has units that are the square of those of the original observations, and can be used for data measured on an interval or ratio scale.

$$s^2 = \frac{1}{n - 1} \sum_{i=1}^{n} (x_i - \bar{x})^2 \qquad (4.3)$$

The variance can be obtained by carrying out the same procedure as for the mean and standard deviation (see above), but this time in the **Descriptives** box (Figure 4.52) click on **Options...** to open the **Descriptives: Options** box. Simply check **Range** in the **Descriptives: Options** box, as shown in Figure 4.61.

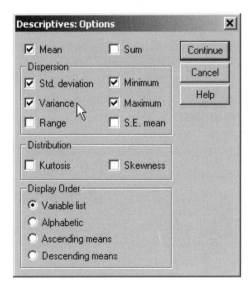

Figure 4.61 The **Descriptives: Options** box – obtaining the variance

Click on **Continue** to return to the **Descriptives** box and then on **OK**. The resulting **Output** is shown in Figure 4.62, in which the value of the variance is given as approximately 317.14 year².

Descriptive Statistics

	N	Minimum	Maximum	Mean	Std. Deviation	Variance
Age of Respondent	1514	18	89	45.63	17.808	317.140
Valid N (listwise)	1514					

Figure 4.62 Output screen showing the value of the variance

DISTRIBUTION SHAPE

DIAGRAMMATIC REPRESENTATION

Histogram

Interval and ratio data can be represented by histograms. Suppose we wish to represent the ratio variable highlighted in Figure 4.50 (the age of respondents in the U.S. General Social Survey) as a histogram. We could select **Histograms** in the **Frequencies: Charts** box shown in Figure 4.10. Alternatively, simply select **Graphs\Histogram...**, as shown in Figure 4.63.

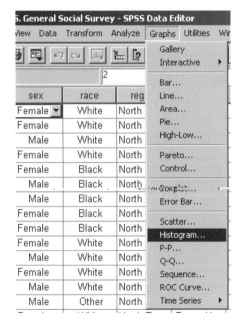

Figure 4.63 Selecting **histogram** from the **Graphs** menu

This opens the **Histogram** box, in which you should select the required variable (see Figure 4.64).

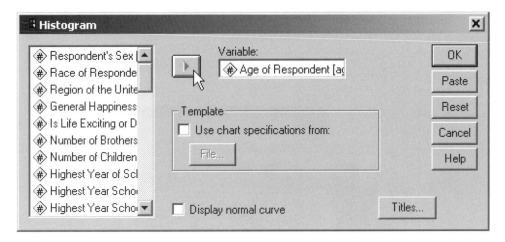

Figure 4.64 The **Histogram** box

Figure 4.64 The **Histogram** box

Click on **OK**. The cut-off points for the intervals in the histogram are chosen automatically. The default histogram produced by SPSS in the **Output** is shown in Figure 4.65.

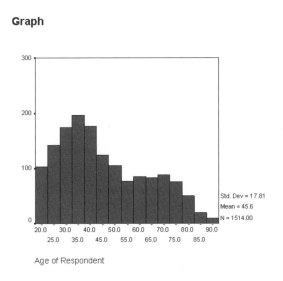

Figure 4.65 Histogram

Scale axis range
You can change the range of a scale axis on a graph such as a histogram as follows. Suppose we are starting with the histogram shown in Figure 4.65 and wish to change

the vertical (ordinate) axis scale range from its current zero to 300 to zero to 200. First double-click on the histogram (in the **Output** screen) to go into edit mode (the SPSS Chart Editor) in the usual way. Now double-click on any of the numbers labelling the vertical axis. This opens the **Scale Axis** box shown in Figure 4.66.

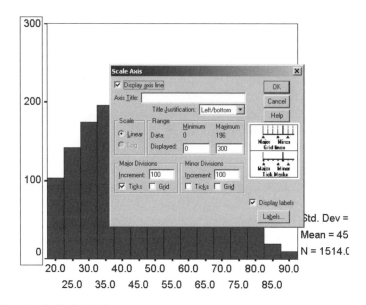

Figure 4.66 Opening the **Scale Axis** box

In the **Range** section of the **Scale Axis** box, change **Maximum** from 300 to 200 (Figure 4.67).

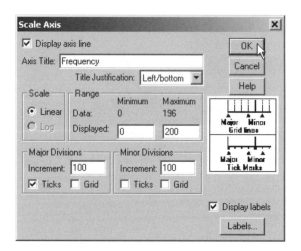

Figure 4.67 Edited Scale Axis box

Clicking **OK** returns you to the Chart Editor, which you should now close. The edited histogram appears in the **Output** window, as shown in Figure 4.68.

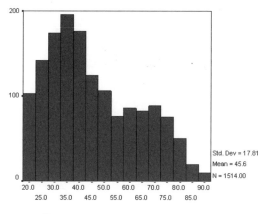

Std. Dev = 17.81
Mean = 45.6
N = 1514.00

Age of Respondent

Figure 4.68 Edited histogram

For a histogram, the menu for editing the cut-off points for intervals is accessed by double-clicking on the horizontal axis in the Chart Editor.

Stem-and-leaf diagram

A stem-and-leaf diagram, which can also be used to represent continuous (interval or ratio) data, differs from a histogram in that it allows all the individual data to be shown. To represent the continuous (ratio) variable highlighted in Figure 4.50 as a stem-and-leaf diagram, first select **Analyze\Descriptive Statistics\Explore...** (Figure 4.69).

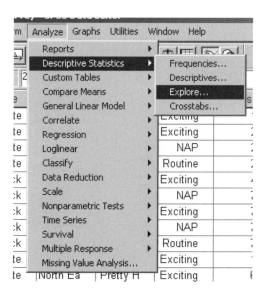

Figure 4.69 Selecting **Explore**

In the resulting **Explore** box, select the required variable and the **Display Plots** radio button, as shown in Figure 4.70.

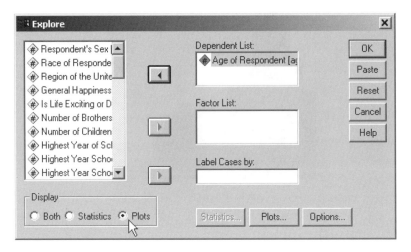

Figure 4.70 The **Explore** box

Boxplots (see below) and stem-and-leaf diagrams are produced by default. (To obtain only boxplots or stem-and-leaf diagrams, click on **Plots...** and then in the resulting **Explore: Plots** box make the appropriate choice.) Clicking **OK** in the Explore box then produces both a boxplot and a stem-and-leaf diagram in the **Output**. The stem-and-leaf diagram is shown in Figure 4.71.

Age of Respondent

```
Age of Respondent Stem-and-Leaf Plot

Frequency    Stem &  Leaf

    12.00      1 .  899
   143.00      2 .  00001111111222222233333344444
   150.00      2 .  55555566666667777778888888899999
   187.00      3 .  0000000111111122222222233333333334444444
   195.00      3 .  5555555555566666667777777788888889999999
   167.00      4 .  00000001111111122222223333333444444
   113.00      4 .  555566777778888889999
    87.00      5 .  000011122223334444
    78.00      5 .  555667778888999
    87.00      6 .  00011112223333444
    84.00      6 .  555566677778888999
    95.00      7 .  0001111222233333444
    53.00      7 .  5566677889
    43.00      8 .  001122234
    20.00      8 .  5799&

Stem width:    10
Each leaf:        5 case(s)


& denotes fractional leaves.
```

Figure 4.71 Stem-and-leaf diagram

Boxplot

The above procedure for a stem-and-leaf diagram also produces a boxplot (box-and-whisker plot) in **Output** (Figure 4.72).

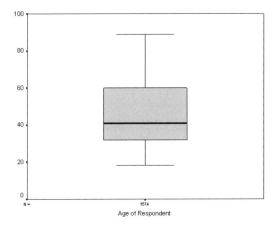

Figure 4.72 Boxplot

In a boxplot the upper and lower boundaries of the box are the upper and lower quartiles, respectively. The box length is the interquartile range. The thick line inside the box is the median. The vertical lines from the box (whiskers) extend to the smallest and largest observations that are less than one interquartile range from the end of the box. O (outlier) marks points outside this range but less than 1.5 interquartile distances away. E marks points more than 1.5 interquartile ranges from the end of the box. There are no points marked O or E in Figure 4.72.

FREQUENCIES

Frequency tables can be obtained as described above (Figures 4.3 to 4.5).

SKEWNESS

Skewness measures the asymmetry of a distribution. Figure 4.73 shows two asymmetric, skewed distributions. Figure 4.73(a) shows a distribution that is negatively skewed, as it contains relatively more large values and relatively few smaller values. In contrast, the distribution shown in Figure 4.73(b) is positively skewed, as it contains relatively more small values and relatively few larger values.

SPSS can calculate a mathematical measure of skewness in which symmetry corresponds to a skewness of zero, and a positive or negative value of skewness corresponds to a positively or negatively skewed distribution, respectively. A normal distribution (see below) is symmetrical about its mean and has a skewness of zero. For a large distribution, a departure from symmetry is taken to exist if the modulus (absolute value) of the skewness is more than 1.96 times the standard error:

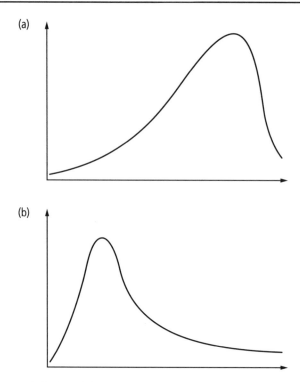

Figure 4.73 (a) A negatively skewed distribution; (b) a positively skewed distribution

For a large sample,
Significant departure from symmetry ⇔
|skewness| > 1.96 (standard error of skewness)

For the data shown in Figure 4.50, the skewness of the age of respondents can be calculated as follows. First obtain the **Descriptives** box by selecting **Analyze\Descriptive Statistics\Descriptives...** (Figures 4.51 and 4.52). In the **Descriptives** box move the required variable (age) into the **Variables** section, and then click **Options...** . In the resulting **Descriptives: Options** box check **Skewness** in the **Distribution** section as shown in Figure 4.74.

Click on **Continue** to return to the **Descriptives** box. Then click on **OK** to obtain the skewness in the **Output**, as shown in Figure 4.75.

This output shows that the distribution has a skewness of +0.524, which is much greater than 1.96 times the standard error (0.063) of the skewness. This is shown as:

$$0.524 \gg 1.96 \, (0.063)$$
$$\approx 0.123$$

Hence the distribution is positively skewed. This is in line with what would be expected from the histogram shown in Figure 4.65 and the boxplot shown in Figure 4.72.

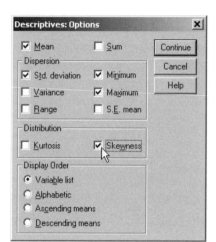

Figure 4.74 Selecting **skewness**

Descriptive Statistics

	N	Minimum	Maximum	Mean	Std.	Skewness	
	Statistic	Statistic	Statistic	Statistic	Statistic	Statistic	Std. Error
Age of Respondent	1514	18	89	45.63	17.808	.524	.063
Valid N (listwise)	1514						

Figure 4.75 Skewness output

KURTOSIS

The kurtosis of a distribution is a calculated value that indicates the pointedness of the shape of that distribution. A positive value for the kurtosis is associated with a more pointed distribution, while a negative value is associated with a flatter distribution. A normal distribution (see below) is associated with a kurtosis of zero. For a large sample, the kurtosis is considered to be significantly different to zero if the following holds.

> For a large sample,
> kurtosis is significantly different from zero
> $\Leftrightarrow$ |kurtosis| > 1.96 (standard error of kurtosis)

The kurtosis of a distribution is obtained in SPSS in a similar manner to the way in which the skewness is obtained. For the data shown in Figure 4.50, the skewness of the age of respondents can be calculated as follows. First obtain the **Descriptives** box by selecting **Analyze\Descriptive Statistics\Descriptives...** (Figures 4.51 and 4.52). In the **Descriptives** box move the required variable (age) into the **Variables** section, and then click **Options...** . In the resulting **Descriptives: Options** box check **Kurtosis** in the **Distribution** section, as shown in Figure 4.76.

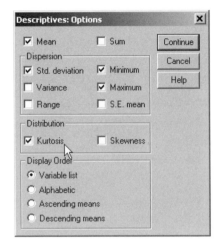

Figure 4.76 Selecting **kurtosis**

Click on **Continue** to return to the **Descriptives** box. Then click on **OK** to obtain the kurtosis in the **Output**, as shown in Figure 4.77.

Descriptive Statistics

	N	Minimum	Maximum	Mean	Std.	Kurtosis	
	Statistic	Statistic	Statistic	Statistic	Statistic	Statistic	Std. Error
Age of Respondent	1514	18	89	45.63	17.808	-.786	.126
Valid N (listwise)	1514						

Figure 4.77 Kurtosis output

This output shows that the distribution has a kurtosis of −0.786, the modulus of which is greater than 1.96 times the standard error (0.126) of the kurtosis. That is,

$$|-0.786| > 1.96 \, (0.126) \approx 0.247$$

Hence the distribution has a significant negative kurtosis. So again, as with the skewness above, the age of respondent distribution appears to differ significantly from a normal distribution on another measure, that of kurtosis. Certainly the histogram shown in Figure 4.65 does not appear to be normal (in the statistical sense of a normal distribution). Formal methods of assessing normality are considered in the following subsection.

NORMAL DISTRIBUTION

Definition
The normal or Gaussian (after Gauss, the mathematician) distribution is a classic bell-shaped distribution which has the appearance shown in Figure 4.78.

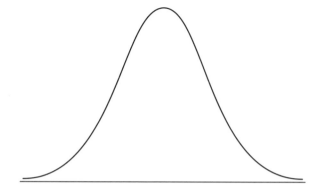

Figure 4.78 The normal distribution

The normal distribution is strictly defined as the probability density function given by:

$$f(x) = \frac{1}{\sigma\sqrt{2\pi}} e^{-\frac{1}{2}\left(\frac{x-\mu}{\sigma}\right)^2}, \qquad x \in \mathbb{R} \qquad (4.4)$$

where μ is the mean

σ is the standard deviation

This distribution (abbreviated to $N(\mu,\sigma^2)$) is standardized to one with a mean (μ) of zero and a variance (σ^2) (and therefore standard deviation, σ) of unity, giving rise to the standard normal distribution $N(0,1)$. The symbol Z is conventionally used for the standard normal variable. The probability density function of the standard normal distribution is therefore given as:

$$f(x) = \frac{1}{\sqrt{2\pi}} e^{-\frac{x^2}{2}}, \qquad x \in \mathbb{R} \qquad (4.5)$$

From Equations 4.4. and 4.5 it can be seen that the (standard) normal distribution is symmetrical about the mean of the distribution, and that the value of $f(x)$ tends to zero as x tends to $\pm \infty$ (plus or minus infinity). These features are shown in Figure 4.79.

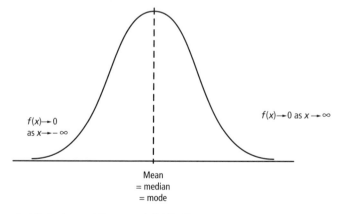

$f(x) \rightarrow 0$ as $x \rightarrow -\infty$

$f(x) \rightarrow 0$ as $x \rightarrow \infty$

Mean
= median
= mode

Figure 4.79 Characteristic features of the normal distribution

Importance of the normal distribution

The normal distribution is of central importance in statistical testing owing to the central limit theorem. Suppose you have a population with overall mean μ and variance σ^2. Now suppose you take n independent and identically distributed random observations from this population, denoted by $X_1, X_2, ..., X_n$, as shown in Figure 4.80. By the central limit theorem, if the number of observations is large (i.e. for large n), the mean of these observations is approximately normal with mean μ and variance σ^2/n. Importantly, this is the case no matter what the underlying distribution of the parent population. (In addition, observations used in statistical tests may often be considered to consist of the means of contributing effects (that are not themselves observed).)

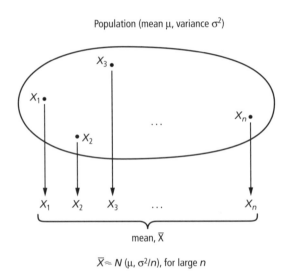

Figure 4.80 Taking n independent and identically distributed random observations from a population

The standard deviation of μ, known as the standard error of μ, is $\sigma/\sqrt{n}$.

Parametric versus non-parametric tests

These are described in Chapter 1. The process of data transformation, to attempt to convert a non-normal distribution into a normal one, is described in the next chapter.

Tests of normality

From the above discussion, and as mentioned in Chapters 1 and 3, it is often important to test whether the sample data come from a normal distribution. Suppose we wish to carry out such a test for the variable (age) highlighted in Figure 4.50. There are three methods that we shall consider.

1. Evaluating the skewness and kurtosis of the data
2. Displaying a normal distribution curve on a histogram of the data
3. Using a probability plot.

1. Skewness and kurtosis

First, we note that both the skewness and kurtosis of the normal distribution are zero. We have seen above how to test whether the skewness and kurtosis of a distribution are significantly different to zero (see Expressions 4.1 and 4.3). If either the skewness or kurtosis is significantly different to zero, then the sample data should usually not be considered to be normal.

2. Displaying the normal curve on a histogram

Second, when plotting histograms, it is possible to ask the program to insert an overlying normal distribution curve which has the mean and variance of the sample data. For example, consider again the histogram for the age of respondents data shown in Figure 4.65. In the **Histograms** box (see above), check the box **Display normal curve**, as shown in Figure 4.81.

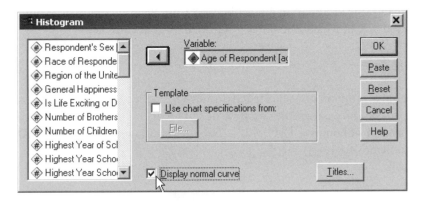

Figure 4.81 The **Histogram** box – displaying a normal curve

Click on **OK** to obtain the histogram with the superimposed normal distribution curve in the **Output** (Figure 4.82).

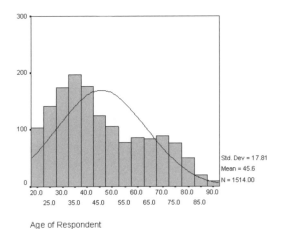

Std. Dev = 17.81
Mean = 45.6
N = 1514.00

Age of Respondent

Figure 4.82 Histogram with superimposed normal curve having the mean and variance of the distribution

It is clear from this graph that the fit between the sample data and a normal distribution is poor.

3. Probability plots

A third option in testing for normality is to utilize probability plots. The n observed data are ordered as follows:

$$x_1 \leq x_2 \leq \ldots \leq x_n$$

n normal quantiles (also known as normal scores), with values $z_1, z_2,\ldots, z_n$, are calculated from:

$$\Phi(z_i) = \frac{i}{n+1}, i = 1, 2, \ldots n \qquad (4.6)$$

The left-hand side of Equation 4.6 is obtained from the probability distribution given in Equation 4.7, in which Z denotes a standard normal variable.

$$\Phi(z) = \rho(Z \leq z) \qquad (4.7)$$

The computer program plots the ordered values $z_1, z_2,\ldots, z_n$, against ordered values $x_1, x_2,\ldots, x_n$, to produce a quantile–quantile or Q-Q plot.

One way of obtaining a Q-Q plot in SPSS is as follows. Select **Graphs\Q-Q...** as shown in Figure 4.83.

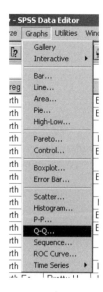

Figure 4.83 Selecting Q-Q plots from the menu

In the resulting **Q-Q Plots** box, move the required variable (age) into the **Variables** section, as shown in Figure 4.84.

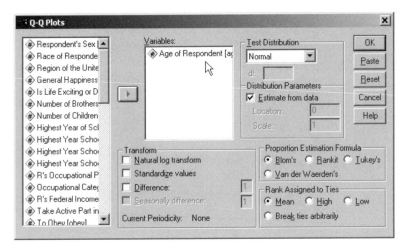

Figure 4.84 The **Q-Q Plots** box

Click on **OK** in the **Q-Q Plots** box. In the **Output** two plots are produced. The Normal Q-Q (Quantile–Quantile) plot shows the observed values of the variable (along the horizontal axis) plotted against the corresponding values predicted if the data are from a standard normal distribution (along the vertical axis). If the data are indeed from a normal distribution, then the points in this plot would be expected to cluster around the straight line (usually produced in the default colour green) shown in Figure 4.85.

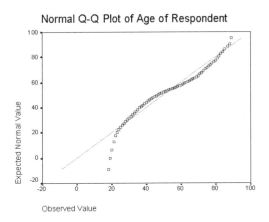

Figure 4.85 Normal Q-Q (Quantile–Quantile) plot

In this case there is a definite deviation from the straight line. The other plot produced is a detrended normal plot. This is a plot of the differences between the observed values and the corresponding predicted values if the sample is from a normal distribution. If the sample is indeed from a normal distribution, then the points should cluster in a horizontal band around zero and there should not be a pattern; this is not the case for the detrended normal Q-Q plot shown in Figure 4.86.

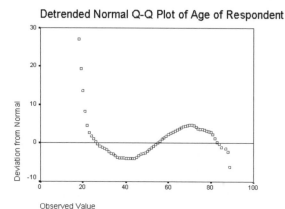

Figure 4.86 Detrended normal Q-Q plot

In this case the distribution should not be taken as having a normal distribution. In such a case, if you wish to use a statistical test requiring the assumption of normality (see Chapter 3), then you may wish to consider using data transformation, as described in the next chapter.

chapter 5

DATA TRANSFORMATION AND SELECTION

DATA TRANSFORMATION

Data transformation involves changing the values of a variable. This may be carried out for a number of reasons, such as correcting coding errors, modifying the coding scheme, creating new variables, constructing an index, or, as seen at the end of the last chapter, in order to alter the distribution of a variable so that it better matches another one, such as the normal distribution. An important feature of SPSS is that there is a choice between transforming an existing variable, or keeping the existing variable and creating a new variable (the transformed one), or choosing not to save the transformation at all (either by opening a new data file or exiting SPSS without saving the transformed variable).

TYPES OF DATA TRANSFORMATION

In SPSS data transformation can be accessed from the Transform menu, as shown in Figure 5.1.

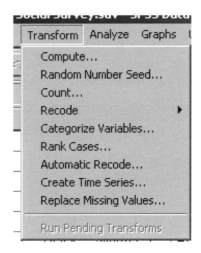

Figure 5.1 Selecting **Transform** from the menu

The following types of data transformation are available:

- Compute – data values are computed according to the formula entered
- Random number seed – this sets the seed used by the pseudo-random number generator to a specific value, so that you can reproduce a sequence of pseudo-random numbers; the random-number seed changes each time SPSS generates a random number for use in transformations
- Count – a new variable is created that for each case how many times specified values occur in other variables
- Recode – discrete values are assigned to a variable (either the same variable or a different variable) based on its current values
- Categorize variables – this converts continuous data into a discrete number of categories
- Rank cases – rank scores are created
- Automatic recode – the consecutive positive integers 1, 2, 3, 4, ... are automatically assigned to a new variable
- Create time series – new time series are created
- Replace missing values – this creates new time series variables from existing ones, replacing missing values with estimates computed with one of several methods.

Descriptions of how to use certain of these transformations follow.

RECODING

In Figure 4.50 in the previous chapter, the continuous variable age represents the age of respondent in the US General Social Survey (supplied with SPSS). Suppose we wish to recode these ages into a separate categorical variable in which the categories are of unequal size: (0 up to but not including 20 years; 20 up to 60 years; and so on). Select **Recode Into Different Variables...**, as shown in Figure 5.2.

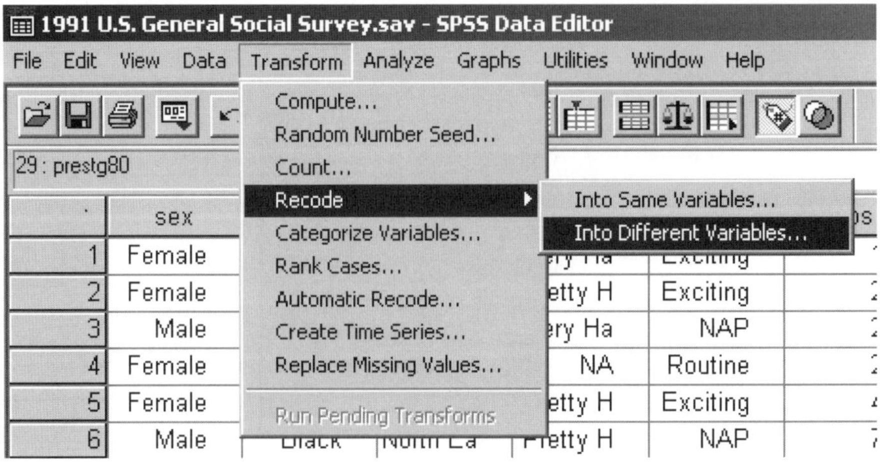

Figure 5.2 Selecting **Recode**

In the resulting **Recode into Different Variables** box, select the required variable (age), type a name for the new categorical variable (ageyrcat, say) into the **Output Variable Name** box, and then click **Change**, as shown in Figure 5.3. (If you wish to give the new variable a label, then simply type that in the **Label** section.)

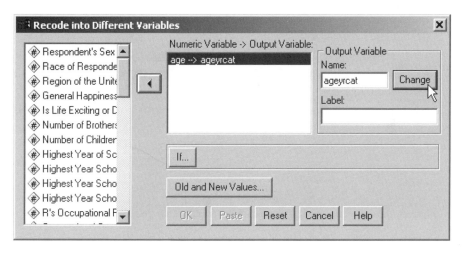

Figure 5.3 The **Recode into Different Variables** box

Next, click **Old and New Values...** to open the **Recode into Different Variables: Old and New Values** box. For the first category, select the **Range** radio button in the **Old Value** group and then enter 0 through 19.999 (for 0 up to 20 years (exclusive)). This will correspond to the category 1, which should therefore be entered in the **New Value** group as shown in Figure 5.4.

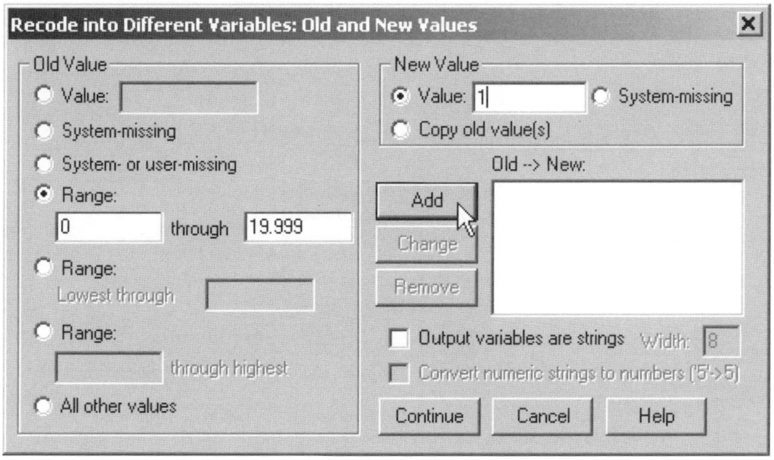

Figure 5.4 The **Recode into Different Variables: Old and New Values** box

Clicking **Add** then results in Figure 5.5.

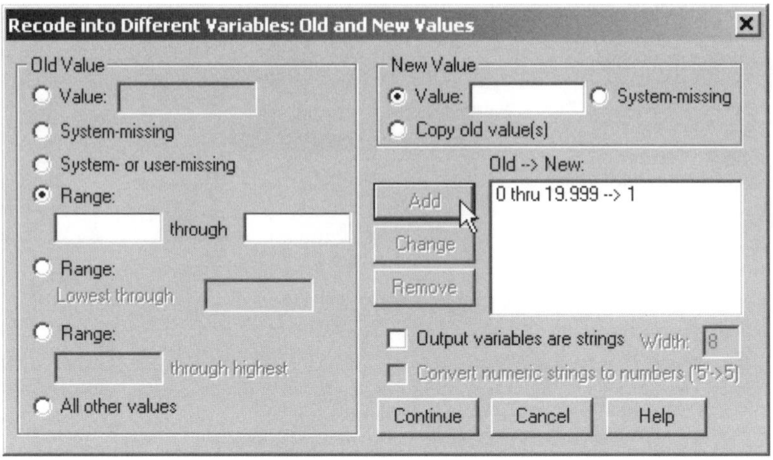

Figure 5.5 Partially completed **Recode into Different Variables: Old and New Values** box

Continue in this way for the other categories, using the appropriate radio button menus. Note that since the original data use 99 for missing values (NA), we must enter this too, in the way shown in Figure 5.6.

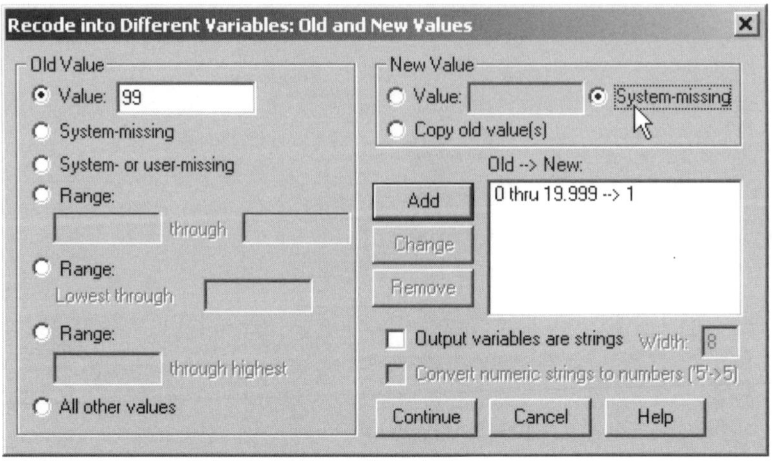

Figure 5.6 Encoding the missing value (99, NA)

The completed box is shown in Figure 5.7.

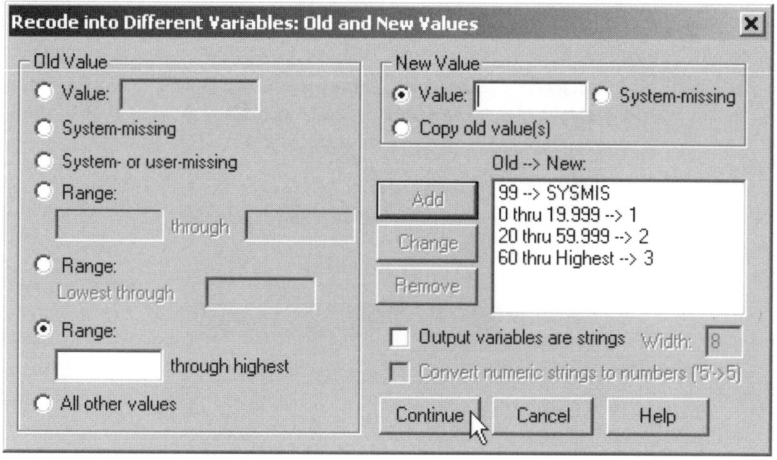

Figure 5.7 Completed **Recode into Different Variables: Old and New Values** box

Click **Continue** to return to the previous box, in which **OK** should be clicked for the data transformation to take place. This can be checked in **Data View** (Figure 5.8).

age	ageyrcat
61	3
32	2
35	2
26	2
25	2
59	2
46	2
NA	.
57	2
64	3
72	3
67	3
33	2
23	2
33	2
59	2
60	3
77	3
52	2

Figure 5.8 Part of **Data View** showing the recoded variable (ageyrcat) and original variable (age)

CATEGORIZING VARIABLES

Suppose this time we wish to convert the ages in the previous example into an ordinal variable consisting of discrete categories of an equal age difference each. This can be achieved more easily by using **Transform\Categorize Variables...** rather than **Transform\Recode**.

Select **Categorize Variables...**, as shown in Figure 5.9.

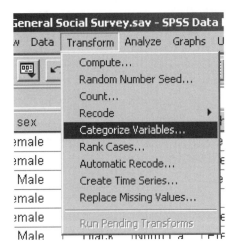

Figure 5.9 Selecting **Categorize Variables**

In the resulting **Categorize Variables** box, select the required variable (age) and type in the required number of categories (4 (by default), say), as shown in Figure 5.10.

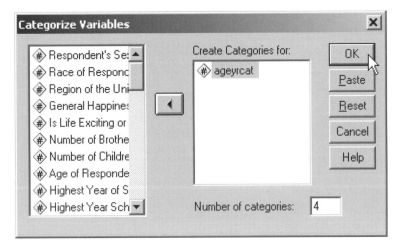

Figure 5.10 The **Categorize Variables** box

Click **OK** for the data transformation to take place. This can be checked in **Data View** (Figure 5.11).

age	nageyrca
61	4
32	2
35	2
26	2
25	2
59	2
46	2
NA	.
57	2
64	4
72	4
67	4
33	2
23	2
33	2
59	2
60	4

Figure 5.11 Part of **Data View** showing the recoded variable (nageyrca) and original variable (age)

COMPUTING VARIABLES

Suppose we wished to convert the ages (in years) in the previous example (age, highlighted in Figure 4.50) into ages expressed as months. We will save the transformed data as a new variable, agemonth. Select **Compute...**, as shown in Figure 5.12.

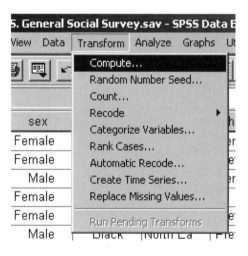

Figure 5.12 Selecting **Compute**

In the resulting **Compute Variable** box, type in the name of the target variable (agemonth), click the **Type&Label** button to make any required modifications to the target variable, and use the **Numeric Expression** part of the box to construct the required formula (using the arrow buttons to paste variables and functions as required). The functions available are shown in the Appendix. The calculator pad operators available are shown in Table 5.1.

Table 5.1 Calculator pad operators

Operator	Function
+	Add
–	Subtract
*	Multiply
/	Divide
**	Raise to power
<	Less than
<=	Less than or equal to
=	Equal to
&	And
~	Not
>	Greater than
>=	Greater than or equal to
–=	Not equal to
		Or
()	Grouping parentheses

In our example, the formula required is agemonth = age*12, as shown in Figure 5.13.

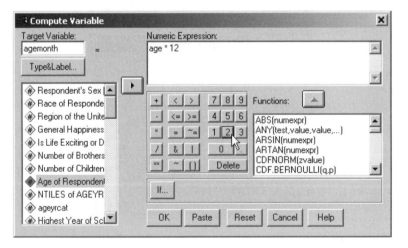

Figure 5.13 The **Compute Variable** box

Click on **OK** for the data transformation to take place. This can be checked in the data file (Figure 5.14).

age	agemonth
61	732
32	384
35	420
26	312
25	300
59	708
46	552
NA	.
57	684
64	768
72	864
67	804
33	396

Figure 5.14 Part of **Data View** showing the computed variable (agemonth) and original variable (age)

Ladder of powers

The compute function is particularly useful for carrying out transformations such as taking the logarithm (LG10 (logarithm to the base 10) or LN (natural logarithm, to the base e)) or square root (SQRT) when trying to make the distribution of a variable more closely match the normal distribution. The following ladder of powers is useful in determining the transformations to try first.

$$\ldots, x^{-2}, x^{-1}, x^{-1/2}, \ln x, x^{1/2}, x^{2}, \ldots$$

For example, if the data distribution has a strong positive skewness, and if the data are themselves all positive, then you need to pull down higher values more than lower values and so you may usefully try the transformations $\ln x$ (the natural logarithm function) and $x^{1/2}$ (the square root function) first. Alternatively, with a strong negative skewness, you should try a function on the right-hand side of the ladder of powers, that is, a squared (x^2) or higher power.

CONDITIONAL TRANSFORMATIONS

If you wish, you can choose to transform only a selected number of cases in a given variable. For instance, in the previous example (age to agemonth) suppose we only wish to transform the ages of males aged over 50 years. To do this, click on the **If...** button in the **Compute Variable** box (Figure 5.13). This opens the box shown in Figure 5.15, which should be completed as shown. The logical operators of the calculator pad, shown in Table 5.1 (<, <=, =, &, ~, >, >=, ~=, |) can be used to build logical operations.

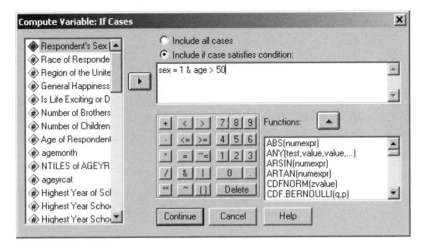

Figure 5.15 **Compute Variable: If Cases** box

Clicking on **Continue** returns you to the **Compute Variable** box, in which clicking **OK** allows the conditional transformation to take place.

DATA SELECTION

In order to use only selected cases, choose **Select Cases...**, as shown in Figure 5.16.

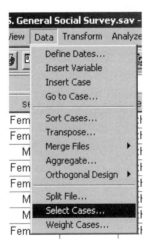

Figure 5.16 Selecting **Select Cases**

This opens the **Select Cases** box. Suppose we wanted to select females aged 30 years or over in the previous example (age; Figure 4.50). In the **Select Cases** box choose the **If condition is satisfied** radio button. If you wish the selection to be temporary, also choose the **Filtered** radio button, while if you wish the selection to be permanent, choose **Deleted**. Then click on the **If...** button shown in Figure 5.17.

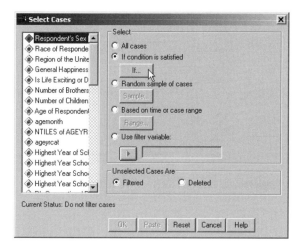

Figure 5.17 The **Select Cases** box

In the next box, construct the required logical operation (Figure 5.18).

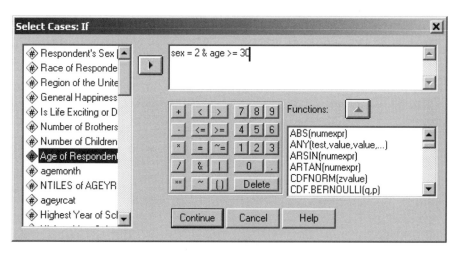

Figure 5.18 The **Select Cases: If** box

Click on **Continue**, and then on **OK** in the **Select Cases** box. The **Data View** confirms that the required selection has been made, with the case numbers of deselected cases being crossed, as shown in Figure 5.19.

	sex	age
1	Female	61
2	Female	32
3	Male	35
4	Female	26
5	Female	25
6	Male	59
7	Male	46
8	Female	NA
9	Female	57
10	Female	64
11	Male	72
12	Female	67
13	Male	33

Figure 5.19 Part of **Data View** showing selected cases

chapter 6

COMPARING TWO
SAMPLE AVERAGES

PARAMETRIC TESTS

The *t*-test is used for testing the null hypothesis that two population means are equal when the variable being investigated has a normal distribution in each population and the population variances are equal. SPSS automatically checks that the variances of the two groups are not significantly different, and if they are the program gives adjusted probabilities corresponding to the value of *t*. Before carrying out a *t*-test, therefore, you should check that the data come from normal distributions (see Chapter 4); it is a useful step to plot the data.

INDEPENDENT SAMPLES *t*-TEST

This procedure tests the null hypothesis that the data are a sample from a population in which the mean of a test variable is equal in two independent (unrelated) groups of cases.

Suppose we wish to test the null hypothesis, at the 5% level of significance, that there is no difference between the population mean ages of the males and females in the data file shown in Figure 6.1.

	age	sex
1	22.9	male
2	23.3	male
3	20.6	male
4	22.3	male
5	22.6	male
6	25.1	male
7	47.8	male
8	32.8	female
9	37.4	male
10	20.8	male
11	43.0	male
12	23.1	male
13	32.3	male

Figure 6.1 Part of a data file showing ages (highlighted) of male and female subjects

First, we confirm that the data come from normal distributions. The procedure for carrying this out is not shown here, as it appears in Chapter 4. In particular, it is worthwhile plotting boxplots (comparing male ages with female ages).

If we wish to plot the ages of each sex with error bars representing the standard error of the mean, first we make the selection shown in Figure 6.2.

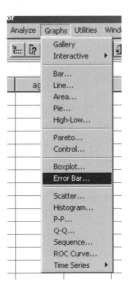

Figure 6.2 Selecting **Error Bar** in **Graphs**

Then press **Define** in the **Error Bar** box (Figure 6.3).

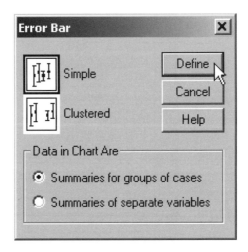

Figure 6.3 The **Error Bar** box

Make the appropriate choices in the dialogue box (Figure 6.4).

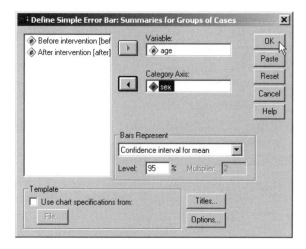

Figure 6.4 The **Define Simple Error Bar: Summaries for Groups of Cases** box

On clicking **OK**, the required plot appears in the **Output**, as shown in Figure 6.5.

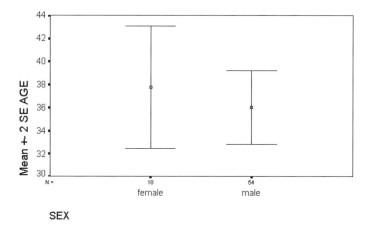

Figure 6.5 The Error Bar plot

The independent (unrelated) samples *t*-test procedure is chosen as shown in Figure 6.6.

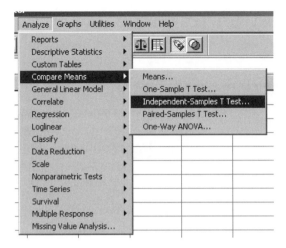

Figure 6.6 Selecting the independent samples *t*-test

The appropriate variable selections are made in the corresponding dialogue box, as shown in Figure 6.7.

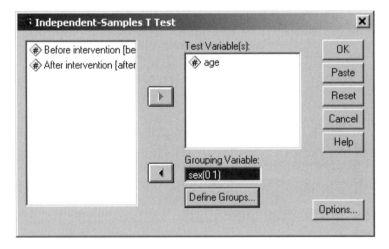

Figure 6.7 The **Independent-Samples T Test** box

(If a confidence interval other than 95 per cent for the difference between the means is required, click on **Options** and make the necessary alteration.) Clicking on **OK** then gives the required results in the **Output** (Figure 6.8). (In this case, the **Output** is shown for a version of SPSS earlier than version 10, in case you are using an early version; the appearance of the version 10 **Output** is shown in Figure 6.18.)

```
t-tests for Independent Samples of SEX
```

Variable	Number of Cases	Mean	SD	SE of Mean
AGE				
fema	18	37.7723	11.295	2.662
male	54	36.0361	11.754	1.600

```
        Mean Difference = 1.7362

        Levene's Test for Equality of Variances: F= .221   P= .640
```

	t-test for Equality of Means				95%
Variances	t-value	df	2-Tail Sig	SE of Diff	CI for Diff
Equal	.55	70	.586	3.169	(−4.585, 8.057)
Unequal	.56	30.23	.580	· 3.106	(−4.605, 8.077)

Figure 6.8 Output screen showing the results of an independent samples *t*-test

From the upper table in Figure 6.8 we can see that for the 18 female subjects, the mean age is 37.7723 years, with a standard deviation of 11.295 years and a standard error of the mean of 2.662 years. The corresponding figures for the 54 male subjects are 36.0361 years, 11.754 years and 1.600 years, respectively. Under this table we are told that the mean difference between the two groups is 1.7362 years.

The program automatically checks if the variances of the two groups are significantly different, using Levene's test. If the variances are *not* significantly different (using the *F* distribution) then the value of the probability adjacent to the value of *F* is greater than the significance level (commonly 5%, that is, 0.05). This is the case here, as shown in the highlighted output area in Figure 6.9.

```
Mean Difference = 1.7362


Levene's Test for Equality of Variances: F= .221    P= .640
```

Figure 6.9 Part of the output screen of Figure 6.8 with Levene's Test for Equality of Variances highlighted

Therefore, in this case, the appropriate results are those in the upper row of the lower table of Figure 6.8 (**Equal Variances**), highlighted in Figure 6.10.

```
        Levene's Test for Equality of Variances: F= .221    P= .640
```

	t-test for Equality of Means				95%
Variances	t-value	df	2-Tail Sig	SE of Diff	CI for Diff
Equal	.55	70	.586	3.169	(−4.585, 8.057)
Unequal	.56	30.23	.580	3.106	(−4.605, 8.077)

Figure 6.10 Part of the output screen of Figure 6.8 with the Equal Variances row of results highlighted

From this row we can see that the value of t is 0.55, which, with 70 degrees of freedom, corresponds to $P = 0.586$ (two-tailed), which is clearly not significant. Hence the ages of the male and female subjects are not significantly different. The 95% confidence interval for the difference between their ages is −4.585 to 8.057 years; this confidence interval includes the value zero, which is consistent with the finding that the ages of the two groups are not significantly different at the 5% level of significance. These findings are also consistent with the initial plot shown in Figure 6.5.

If Levine's test had shown that the variances were significantly different, then the second row (**Unequal Variances**) in Figure 6.10 would have been used instead.

PAIRED SAMPLES *t*-TEST

This procedure tests the null hypothesis that two population means are equal when the observations for the two groups can be paired in some way. For example, cases may consist of patients observed before and after an intervention, thereby giving rise to pairs of data. Pairing (a repeated measures or within-subjects design) is used to make the two groups as similar as possible, allowing differences observed between the two groups to be attributed more readily to the variable of interest.

Figure 6.11 shows the diastolic blood pressures (in mmHg: millimetres of mercury) of 12 men before and after a particular treatment.

1 : before		78
	before	after
1	78	76
2	86	80
3	84	86
4	82	80
5	94	88
6	80	78
7	86	78
8	76	78
9	92	88
10	88	84
11	86	80
12	80	80
13		

Figure 6.11 Part of a data file showing diastolic blood pressures of 12 male subjects before and after a certain treatment

Before running the paired samples *t*-test procedure, it is useful to plot the paired data as a scatterplot (scatter diagram or dot graph) by making the selection shown in Figure 6.12.

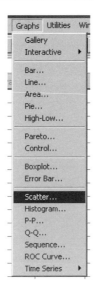

Figure 6.12 Selecting **Scatter** in **Graphs**

In the **Scatterplot** box choose the default **Simple** type of scatter diagram, and click **Define** (Figure 6.13).

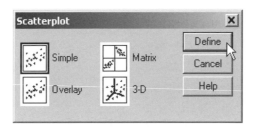

Figure 6.13 The **Scatterplot** box

In the next dialogue box select the two paired variables (Figure 6.14).

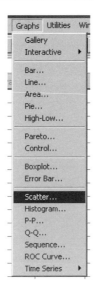

Figure 6.14 The **Simple Scatterplot** box

On clicking **OK**, the required plot appears in the **Output**, as shown in Figure 6.15.

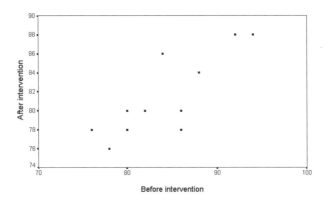

Figure 6.15 Scatterplot of the data file of Figure 6.11

With paired data, scatterplots allow anomalies in the data set to be checked for. In this case there are clearly no obvious outliers.

The paired (related) samples *t*-test procedure is chosen, as shown in Figure 6.16.

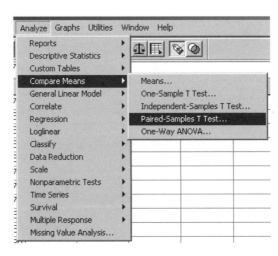

Figure 6.16 Selecting the paired samples *t*-test

The appropriate paired variable selection is made in the corresponding dialogue box, as shown in Figure 6.17.

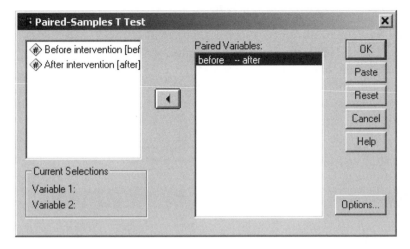

Figure 6.17 The **Paired-Samples T Test** box

(If a confidence interval other than 95% for the difference between the means is required, click on **Options** and make the necessary alteration.) Clicking on **OK** then gives the required results in the **Output** (Figure 6.18; SPSS version 10 output).

Paired Samples Statistics

		Mean	N	Std. Deviation	Std. Error Mean
Pair 1	Before intervention	84.33	12	5.449	1.573
	After intervention	81.33	12	4.119	1.189

Paired Samples Correlations

		N	Correlation	Sig.
Pair 1	Before intervention & After intervention	12	.805	.002

Paired Samples Test

		Paired Differences							
					95% Confidence Interval of the Difference				
		Mean	Std. Deviation	Std. Error Mean	Lower	Upper	t	df	Sig. (2-tailed)
Pair 1	Before intervention - After intervention	3.00	3.247	.937	.94	5.06	3.200	11	.008

Figure 6.18 Output screen showing the results of a paired samples *t*-test

From the upper part of Figure 6.18 we can see that the mean diastolic blood pressure after the intervention is 81.33 mmHg, with a standard deviation of 4.119 mmHg, while before the intervention the corresponding figures are 84.33 and 5.449 mmHg, respectively. The correlation coefficient (see Chapter 9) for the 12 pairs of observations is 0.805 (with an associated two-tailed significance value of 0.002). From the lower part of Figure 6.18 we can see that the mean difference between the two groups is 3.00 mmHg (that is, the diastolic blood pressure is on average 3 mmHg *lower* after the intervention), with a standard deviation of 3.247 mmHg. The value of *t* is 3.20, which, on 11 degrees of freedom, corresponds to $P = 0.008$ (two-tailed), which is clearly significant. Hence the diastolic blood pressure after the intervention is significantly lower than that before the intervention ($P = 0.008$). The 95% confidence interval for the difference is 0.94 to 5.06 mmHg; this confidence interval does not include the value zero, which is consistent with the finding that the ages of the two groups are significantly different at the 5% level of significance.

If you wish to see more significant figures for a value given in the **Output**, simply double-click on the appropriate figure.

NONPARAMETRIC TESTS

For data that do not fulfil the criteria for using parametric tests, SPSS offers nonparametric tests. As mentioned earlier in this book, note that nonparametric tests should not be used in preference if the data do fulfil the criteria for using parametric tests, since the nonparametric tests are less powerful, in a statistical sense, than their nonparametric equivalents.

INDEPENDENT SAMPLES

The Mann–Whitney U test is an alternative to the independent samples *t*-test, in which the actual data values are replaced by ranks for the calculations.

Let us test the null hypothesis, at the 5% level of significance, that there is no difference between the population mean ages of the males and females in the US General Social Survey data (supplied with SPSS). Tests of normality (not shown here) show that the data are not from normal distributions. Once again, we plot the data (not shown). Rather than trying to transform the data, in this case we choose non-parametric testing.

The Mann–Whitney U test is chosen as shown in Figure 6.19.

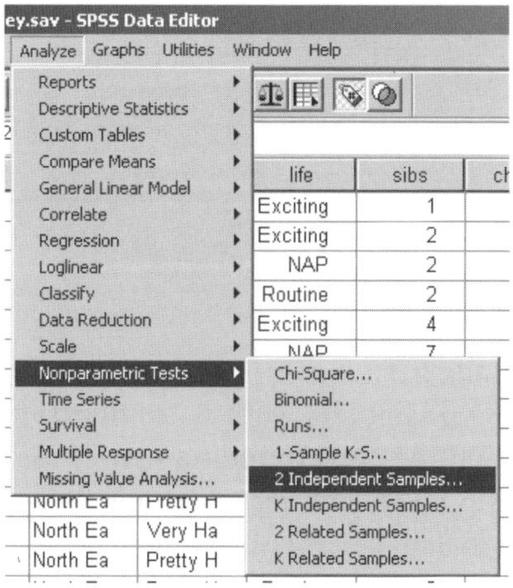

Figure 6.19 Selecting **Nonparametric Tests: 2 Independent Samples**

The appropriate variable selections are made in the corresponding dialogue box, as shown in Figure 6.20.

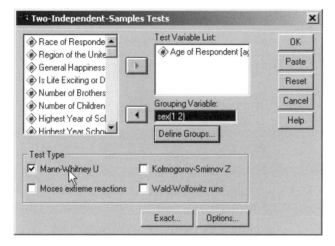

Figure 6.20 The **Two-Independent-Samples Tests** box

Clicking on **OK** then gives the required results in the **Output** (Figure 6.21).

Mann-Whitney Test

Ranks

	Respondent's Sex	N	Mean Rank	Sum of Ranks
Age of Respondent	Male	636	726.92	462319.53
	Female	878	779.65	684535.50
	Total	1514		

Test Statistics[a]

	Age of Respondent
Mann-Whitney U	259753.500
Wilcoxon W	462319.500
Z	-2.317
Asymp. Sig. (2-tailed)	.021

a. Grouping Variable: Respondent's Sex

Figure 6.21 Output screen showing the results of a Mann–Whitney U test

From this **Output** we can see that there is a significant difference between the ages of the male and female subjects according to this nonparametric test ($P = 0.021$ (two-tailed)).

PAIRED (RELATED) SAMPLES

Let us return again to the example of testing the null hypothesis that there is no difference between the diastolic blood pressures of 12 men before and after a particular treatment, for the dataset shown in Figure 6.11. The scatterplot for these data has already been plotted (Figure 6.15).

The nonparametric tests for paired (two related) samples are selected as shown in Figure 6.22.

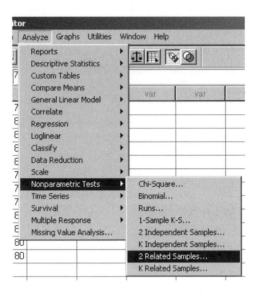

Figure 6.22 Selecting the nonparametric tests for paired (two related) samples

The appropriate paired variable selection is made in the corresponding dialogue box, as shown in Figure 6.23.

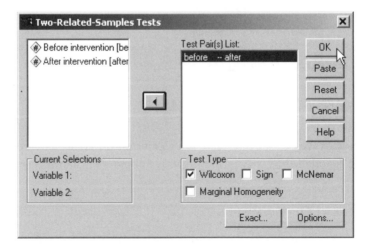

Figure 6.23 The **Two-Related-Samples Tests** box

Three nonparametric tests are offered:

- The Sign test is based on the directions of the differences between two variables.
- The Wilcoxon signed rank test makes no assumptions about the shapes of the distribution of the two variables. The absolute values of the differences between the two variables are calculated for each case and ranked from smallest to largest. The test statistic is based on the sums of ranks for negative and positive differences. It is more powerful, statistically, than the Sign test.
- McNemar's test is used to determine changes in proportions for related samples. It is often used for 'before and after' experimental designs when the dependent variable is dichotomous.

Since our data are not dichotomous, we have a choice between the first two, and will choose the more powerful test, namely the Wilcoxon test. This has been chosen (by default) in Figure 6.23. Clicking on **OK** then gives the required results in the **Output** (Figure 6.24).

Wilcoxon Signed Ranks Test

Ranks

		N	Mean Rank	Sum of Ranks
After intervention - Before intervention	Negative Ranks	9[a]	6.67	60.00
	Positive Ranks	2[b]	3.00	6.00
	Ties	1[c]		
	Total	12		

a. After intervention < Before intervention
b. After intervention > Before intervention
c. Before intervention = After intervention

Test Statistics[b]

	After intervention - Before intervention
Z	-2.431[a]
Asymp. Sig. (2-tailed)	.015

a. Based on positive ranks.
b. Wilcoxon Signed Ranks Test

Figure 6.24 Output screen showing the results of a Wilcoxon signed rank test

From this **Output** we see that according to this nonparametric test the diastolic blood pressure after the intervention is significantly lower than that before the intervention ($P = 0.015$ (two-tailed)).

chapter 7

CONTINGENCY TABLES

DEFINITION

A contingency table, referred to as a crosstabulation in SPSS, is a table with a cell for every combination of values of two or more variables. The table shows the number of cases having each specific combination of values.

A contingency table with r rows and c columns is referred to as a $r \times c$ contingency table. Note that in counting the number of rows and columns, variable labels and marginal totals are not taken into account. For example, the core of a hypothetical 4×2 contingency table is shown in Figure 7.1.

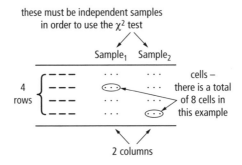

Figure 7.1 The core structure of a 4×2 contingency table. Based on Puri BK and Tyrer P (1992) *Sciences Basic to Psychiatry*, with permission from Churchill Livingstone, Edinburgh

Figure 7.1 can be expanded by adding in the marginal totals (Figure 7.2); this does not alter the number of rows (4) or number of columns (2).

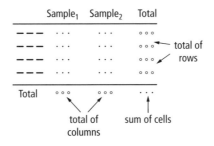

Figure 7.2 A 4×2 contingency table with added marginal totals. Based on Puri BK and Tyrer P (1992) *Sciences Basic to Psychiatry*, with permission from Churchill Livingstone, Edinburgh

CONDITIONS

In this chapter we describe how to compare independent unrelated categorical data presented in the form of contingency tables. The general conditions for using the tests described are:

- the data are categorical, that is, either nominal (qualitative) or ordinal (assigned to ordered categories)
- the actual values of the data, that is, their frequencies, should be used in the contingency tables; proportions, including percentages, should not be used
- the variables should be independent and unrelated
- the parent populations of the samples compared do not have to have any particular distribution; the tests described are non-parametric.

Further conditions for the use of the chi-squared test are given in the next section.

CHI-SQUARED TEST

The chi-squared (χ^2) test is used to test the hypothesis that the row and column variables of a contingency table are independent. The chi-squared statistic is calculated as follows.

$$\chi^2 = \sum_{i=1}^{rc} \frac{(O_i - E_i)^2}{E_i} \tag{7.1}$$

where r = number of rows
c = number of columns
O_i = observed frequencies
E_i = expected frequencies, given by:
$$E_i = \frac{\text{(row total) (column total)}}{\text{overall total}}$$

The number of degrees of freedom of a contingency table is given by (number of rows − 1) × (number of columns − 1). So, a 2 × 2 table has one degree of freedom.

In addition to the general conditions given above, the following criteria should be fulfilled for the chi-squared test to be valid for a contingency table with more than one degree of freedom:

- each expected value > 1
- in at least 80% of cases, expected value > 5

SPSS automatically notes whether or not these criteria are fulfilled when using the chi-squared test.

Figure 7.3 shows part of the **Data View** from the US General Social Survey (supplied with SPSS), in which the sex and race of subjects are highlighted. We shall

	sex	race
1	Female ▼	White
2	Female	White
3	Male	White
4	Female	White
5	Female	Black
6	Male	Black
7	Male	Black
8	Female	Black
9	Female	Black
10	Female	White
11	Male	White
12	Female	White
13	Male	White
14	Male	Other
15	Female	White
16	Female	White
17	Male	White
18	Male	White
19	Female	Black

Figure 7.3 Part of the US General Social Survey Data View, with sex and race highlighted

test the null hypothesis that these two variables are independent using the chi-squared test.

Crosstabs (for crosstabulation) is selected, as shown in Figure 7.4.

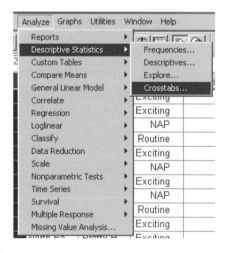

Figure 7.4 Selecting **Crosstabs**

In the resulting **Crosstabs** box the required variables are selected, as shown in Figure 7.5.

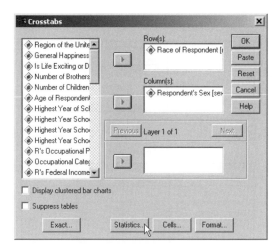

Figure 7.5 The **Crosstabs** box

Click on **Statistics...** and in the resulting **Crosstabs: Statistics** box select **Chi-square** (Figure 7.6).

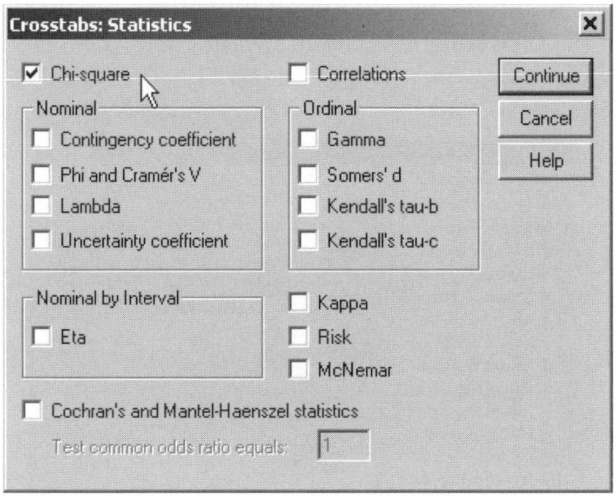

Figure 7.6 The **Crosstabs: Statistics** box

Click on **Continue** to return to the **Crosstabs** box. Clicking on **OK** then takes you to the **Output** screen with the results of the chi-squared analysis, shown in Figure 7.7.

Race of Respondent * Respondent's Sex Crosstabulation

Count

		Respondent's Sex		Total
		Male	Female	
Race of Respondent	White	545	719	1264
	Black	71	133	204
	Other	20	29	49
Total		636	881	1517

Chi-Square Tests

	Value	df	Asymp. Sig. (2-sided)
Pearson Chi-Square	5.011[a]	2	.082
Likelihood Ratio	5.094	2	.078
Linear-by-Linear Association	2.944	1	.086
N of Valid Cases	1517		

a. 0 cells (.0%) have expected count less than 5. The minimum expected count is 20.54.

Figure 7.7 Output screen showing the results of a chi-squared test

From this **Output** we can see that the value of chi-squared (appearing in the row labelled **Pearson Chi-Square**) is 5.011, with 2 degrees of freedom (because this is a 2×3 table). This is not significant ($P = 0.082$) and so the null hypothesis, that the variables sex and race are independent, cannot be rejected.

It is often useful to look at the frequency values which would be expected under the null hypothesis. These can be included in an output table. This option is chosen by clicking **Cells...** in the **Crosstabs** box, as shown in Figure 7.8.

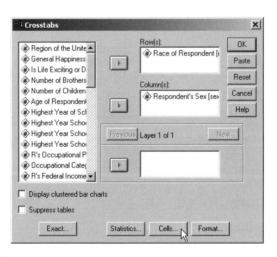

Figure 7.8 Selecting **Cells...** in the **Crosstabs** box

In the resulting box select **Expected**, as shown in Figure 7.9.

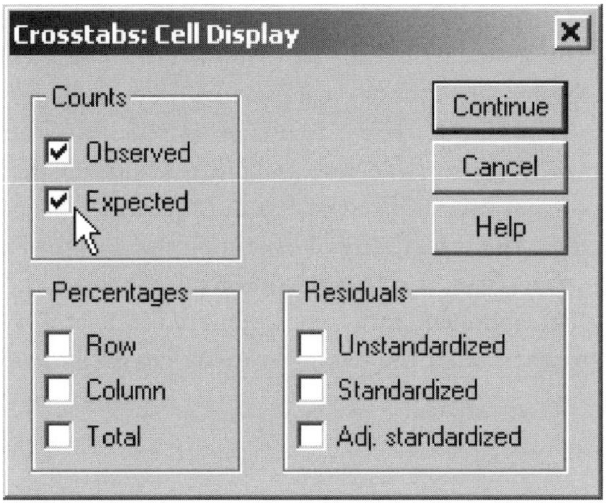

Figure 7.9 The Crosstabs: Cell Display box

Click on **Continue** to return to the **Crosstabs** box. Clicking on **OK** takes you to the **Output** screen with the results of the chi-squared analysis, but this time the table appears as shown in Figure 7.10.

Race of Respondent * Respondent's Sex Crosstabulation

| | | | Respondent's Sex | | Total |
			Male	Female	
Race of Respondent	White	Count	545	719	1264
		Expected Count	529.9	734.1	1264.0
	Black	Count	71	133	204
		Expected Count	85.5	118.5	204.0
	Other	Count	20	29	49
		Expected Count	20.5	28.5	49.0
Total		Count	636	881	1517
		Expected Count	636.0	881.0	1517.0

Figure 7.10 Contingency table in **Output** including both observed and expected frequencies

In each cell the upper figure is the actual observed count, while the lower figure is the frequency expected under the null hypothesis.

FISHER'S EXACT TEST

Fisher's exact probability test is a test for independence in a 2×2 table. It determines the exact probability of obtaining the observed result or one more extreme, if the two variables are independent and the marginal totals are fixed.

SPSS checks if it is dealing with a 2 × 2 table, in which case Fisher's exact probability test is one of the tests carried out by default. For example, if in the previous example we recode the variable race (see Chapter 5 for details of how to carry out this type of data transformation), so that it is dichotomized into white and non-white, then this time running a chi-squared test as before results in the output shown in Figure 7.11. Fisher's exact probability test has automatically been carried out, from which it can be seen that the probability of obtaining the observed result or one more extreme, according to this test, is 0.036 (two-tailed). (You can see that this result is almost the same as that obtained from the chi-squared test, of $P = 0.035$.) Therefore we reject the null hypothesis that the two groups studied are independent.

Race of Respondent * Respondent's Sex Crosstabulation

Count

		Respondent's Sex		Total
		Male	Female	
Race of Respondent	White	545	719	1264
	Non-white	91	162	253
Total		636	881	1517

Chi-Square Tests

	Value	df	Asymp. Sig. (2-sided)	Exact Sig. (2-sided)	Exact Sig. (1-sided)
Pearson Chi-Square	4.425b	1	.035		
Continuity Correction a	4.136	1	.042		
Likelihood Ratio	4.482	1	.034		
Fisher's Exact Test				.036	.021
Linear-by-Linear Association	4.422	1	.035		
N of Valid Cases	1517				

a. Computed only for a 2x2 table

b. 0 cells (.0%) have expected count less than 5. The minimum expected count is 106.07.

Figure 7.11 Output screen showing the results of an analysis using Fisher's exact test

ENTERING A CONTINGENCY TABLE

In the above examples the contingency tables shown in the **Output** screens have been produced by SPSS on the basis of the raw data in the corresponding data files. Sometimes, however, you may wish to analyze a completed contingency table without having to enter all its raw data. Furthermore, sometimes the raw data may not be available. For example, you may wish to check the results of a published contingency table, such as that shown in Table 7.1, which shows the orientation (clockwise or anti-clockwise) of the parietal scalp hair whorl in two groups of people (patients with schizophrenia and normal controls).

Table 7.1 Parietal hair whorl orientation in schizophrenia. (From Puri, BK *et al* (1995) Parietal scalp hair whorl patterns in schizophrenia. *Biological Psychiatry*, **37**, 278–9.)

	Clockwise	Anticlockwise
Schizophrenic patients	114	12
(*n* = 126)	(90.5%)	(9.6%)
Normal controls	1629	261
n = 890	(86.2%)	(13.8%)

These data can be entered directly as a data file in the form shown in Figure 7.12.

	subjects	whorl	count	var
1	schizophrenic	clockwise	114	
2	schizophrenic	anticlockwise	12	
3	normal control	clockwise	1629	
4	normal control	anticlockwise	261	
5				

Figure 7.12 Entering the data of the contingency table shown in Table 7.1 directly into a data file

The first two variables in this data file represent the rows and columns of the contingency table, while the third variable represents the frequencies (count) for each corresponding cell of the table. In order that SPSS treats the last column (count) as one that contains the cell frequencies, the **Weight Cases** box is selected, as shown in Figure 7.13.

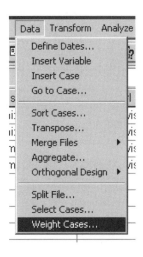

Figure 7.13 Selecting the **Weight Cases** box

In the **Weight Cases** box, make the selection shown in Figure 7.14, thereby informing SPSS that there is a frequency variable (count) by which cases should be weighted.

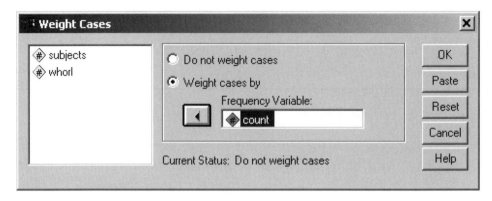

Figure 7.14 The **Weight Cases** box

Click **OK**, and then proceed to carry out the analysis as described earlier in this chapter. The resulting **Output** is shown in Figure 7.15.

SUBJECTS * WHORL Crosstabulation

Count

		WHORL		Total
		clockwise	anticlockwise	
SUBJECTS	schizophrenic	114	12	126
	normal control	1629	261	1890
Total		1743	273	2016

Chi-Square Tests

	Value	df	Asymp. Sig. (2-sided)	Exact Sig. (2-sided)	Exact Sig. (1-sided)
Pearson Chi-Square	1.853[b]	1	.173		
Continuity Correction[a]	1.505	1	.220		
Likelihood Ratio	2.024	1	.155		
Fisher's Exact Test				.225	.107
Linear-by-Linear Association	1.852	1	.174		
N of Valid Cases	2016				

a. Computed only for a 2x2 table

b. 0 cells (.0%) have expected count less than 5. The minimum expected count is 17.06.

Figure 7.15 Output based on the data of Table 7.1

From this **Output** it can be seen that the value of chi-squared for Table 7.1 is 1.853. On one degree of freedom, this is not significant ($P = 0.173$), and so we cannot reject the null hypothesis that there is no statistically significant difference between the two groups.

chapter 8

ANALYSIS OF VARIANCE

Analysis of variance, usually abbreviated to ANOVA, is a method of testing the null hypothesis that several group means are equal in the population, by comparing the sample variance estimated from the group means to that estimated within the groups. In this chapter the application of the following three types of ANOVA using SPSS are described:

- one-way ANOVA
- simple factorial ANOVA
- repeated measures ANOVA.

ONE-WAY ANOVA

This procedure tests the null hypothesis that the data are a sample from a population in which the mean of a test variable is equal in several independent groups of cases defined by a single grouping variable. The 'one-way' in its name comes from the fact that the cases are allocated to the independent groups on the basis of values for that one test variable. There are no repeated measures.

PARAMETRIC TEST

This is a generalization of the independent samples t-test (see Chapter 6). Indeed, when using one-way ANOVA to compare two groups, the results obtained are the same as when an independent samples t-test is carried out. It is important not to substitute the carrying out of multiple t-tests to compare each pair of sample means for an ANOVA; the former procedure would greatly increase the chance that a significant difference will falsely be found.

Assumptions
The assumptions made include the following.

- The data are measured on a ratio or interval scale. If the data are ordinal, then a non-parametric test should be carried out instead, as described below.
- Each group is an independent random sample. If the data contain repeated measures, then a repeated measures ANOVA, described later in this chapter, should be used instead.
- Each group comes from a normally distributed population. This assumption should be checked as described in Chapter 4. If the data are not normal, then it may be possible to make them so by data transformation using an appropriate function

from the ladder of powers described in Chapter 5. If this does not work, then a non-parametric ANOVA can be used instead, as described later in the present chapter.

- The population variances are equal. This assumption can be checked by carrying out a test of homogeneity of variance (using the Levene test of equality of variance). Alternatively, since the one-way ANOVA is fairly robust to small deviations from this assumption, boxplots can be produced, as described in Chapter 4, and the spread of the groups can thereby be checked. (It is, in any case, always good practice to plot the data first before analyzing them.) If there is marked heterogeneity of variance, then a non-parametric ANOVA can be used instead, as described later in this chapter.

Procedure

Table 8.1 shows the plasticity, in arbitrary units, of a group of five independent random samples of each of three different materials, A, B and C. The question to be answered is whether the plasticities of the materials differ.

Table 8.1 Plasticity of three materials, A to C. Based on Puri, BK (1996) *Statistics for the Health Sciences*, with permission from WB Saunders, London

A	13	14	15	14	16
B	16	13	12	11	13
C	14	10	11	13	15

The data have been entered into a data file, as shown in Figure 8.1.

	plasticy	material	
1	13	A	
2	14	A	
3	15	A	
4	14	A	
5	16	A	
6	16	B	
7	13	B	
8	12	B	
9	11	B	
10	13	B	
11	14	C	
12	10	C	
13	11	C	
14	13	C	
15	15	C	
16			

Figure 8.1 The data of Table 8.1 in **Data View**

The one-way ANOVA procedure is selected as shown in Figure 8.2.

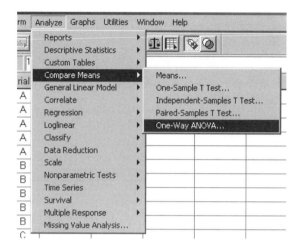

Figure 8.2 Selecting **One-way ANOVA**

The **One-way ANOVA** box is completed as shown in Figure 8.3.

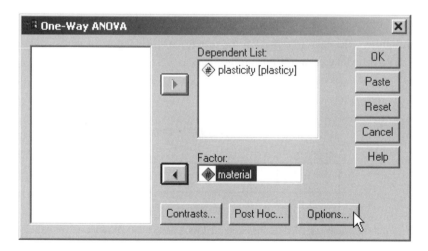

Figure 8.3 The **One-way ANOVA** box

Click the **Options...** button to obtain the **One-way ANOVA: Options** box (see Figure 8.4), in which **Descriptive** can be selected, to give the descriptive statistics for the data, and **Homogeneity-of-variance** can be selected to carry out the Levine test for homogeneity of variances.

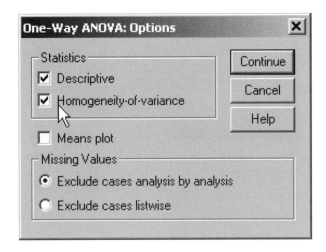

Figure 8.4 The **One-way ANOVA: Options** box

Click **Continue** to return to the **One-way ANOVA** box, and then click **OK**. The Output has three components, in the following order:

- descriptive statistics
- the Levine test for homogeneity of variances
- the ANOVA table.

Figure 8.5 shows the result of the Levine test for homogeneity of variances, with the two-tailed significance probability highlighted.

Test of Homogeneity of Variances

plasticity

Levene Statistic	df1	df2	Sig.
.867	2	12	.445

Figure 8.5 Output from One-way ANOVA: the Levine test for homogeneity of variances (with the two-tailed significance probability highlighted)

It can be seen that the value of this probability is 0.445, which means that the variances can be taken as not being significantly different.

Figure 8.6 shows the result of the ANOVA, with the value of F being 1.473 on 2, 12 degrees of freedom.

ANOVA

plasticity

	Sum of Squares	df	Mean Square	F	Sig.
Between Groups	8.933	2	4.467	1.473	.268
Within Groups	36.400	12	3.033		
Total	45.333	14			

Figure 8.6 Output from One-way ANOVA: the result of the ANOVA (with the value of *F* and its corresponding probability highlighted)

From the table in Figure 8.6 it can be seen that $F(2,12)$ corresponds to a probability of 0.268, which means that the null hypothesis, that the population means are not different, cannot be rejected. Note that an ANOVA ('sums of squares') table is produced as shown in Table 8.2.

Table 8.2 An ANOVA table

Source of variation	Sum of squares	Degree of freedom (*df*)	Mean square	*F*	*P*
Between groups (Treatment)	Explained sum of squares (ESS)	$k - 1$	$ESS/(k - 1)$	$\dfrac{ESS/(k - 1)}{RSS/(n - k)}$	$P(F \geq$ variance ratio)
Within groups (Residual)	Residual sum of squares (RSS)	$n - k$	$RSS/(n - k)$		
Total	Total sum of squares (TSS)	$n - 1$			

The sources of variation appear in the first column. In turn, these are:

- the between groups or 'treatment' source of variation; the number of 'treatments' is denoted by k, and so in our example $k = 3$
- the within groups or 'residual' source of variation
- the total; this is denoted by n and so in our example $n = 15$.

The second column gives the calculated sums of squares. The between groups or explained sum of squares (*ESS*) is given by:

$$ESS = \sum_{j=1}^{k} n_j (\overline{Y}_j - \overline{Y})^2 \tag{8.1}$$

The within groups or residual sum of squares (*RSS*) is given by:

$$RSS = \sum_{j=1}^{k} \sum_{i=1}^{n_j} (Y_{ij} - Y_j)^2 \tag{8.2}$$

The total sum of squares (TSS) is given by:

$$TSS = \sum_{j=1}^{k} \sum_{i=1}^{n_j} (Y_{ij} - \overline{Y})^2 \tag{8.3}$$

In the days before computer programs such as SPSS, when sums of squares were calculated manually, one could make use of the relationship:

$$ESS + RSS = TSS \tag{8.4}$$

The degrees of freedom for sums of squares are shown in the third column. Since there are k treatments, and the formula in Equation (8.1) contains the mean value, one degree of freedom is lost; this corresponds to $(k - 1)$ degrees of freedom. (This is rather similar to the situation that occurs in the calculation of the variance and the standard deviation, in which we also lose one degree of freedom and therefore divide by $(n - 1)$ rather than by n in averaging the squared differences of data values from the mean.) Similarly, the formula in Equation (8.3) also implies the loss of one degree of freedom, the total sum of squares for n observations therefore having $(n - 1)$ degrees of freedom. Finally, the degrees of freedom for the residual sum of squares is found by subtracting $(k - 1)$ from $(n - 1)$. In the fourth column, the mean squares for the first two rows are calculated by dividing the corresponding sums of squares by their respective degrees of freedom. In the fifth column, the variance ratio is calculated using:

$$\text{variance ratio} = \frac{ESS/(k - 1)}{RSS/(n - k)} \tag{8.5}$$

Finally, the last column gives the significance probability corresponding to a value of the F statistic equal to the variance ratio, on $(k - 1, n - k)$ degrees of freedom.

Figure 8.7 shows the descriptive statistics.

Descriptives

plasticity

	N	Mean	Std. Deviation	Std. Error	95% Confidence Interval for Mean		Minimum	Maximum
					Lower Bound	Upper Bound		
A	5	14.40	1.140	.510	12.98	15.82	13	16
B	5	13.00	1.871	.837	10.68	15.32	11	16
C	5	12.60	2.074	.927	10.03	15.17	10	15
Total	15	13.33	1.799	.465	12.34	14.33	10	16

Figure 8.7 Output from One-way ANOVA: the descriptive statistics

Multiple comparisons

While a one-way ANOVA resulting in a statistically significant value of F allows the null hypothesis (that the population means are equal) to be rejected, it does not indicate which means are significantly different. In order to determine this, a multiple comparisons procedure needs to be carried out, either unplanned after it is known that the value of F is statistically significant (*post hoc*) or planned before the value of F is determined (*a priori*). As mentioned above, multiple t-tests comparing each pair of sample means should not be carried out, as this would greatly increase the chance that a significant difference will falsely be found.

A multiple comparison test can be chosen by clicking the **Post Hoc...** button in the **One-Way ANOVA** box (see Figure 8.3) and selecting an appropriate test from the options available shown in Figure 8.8.

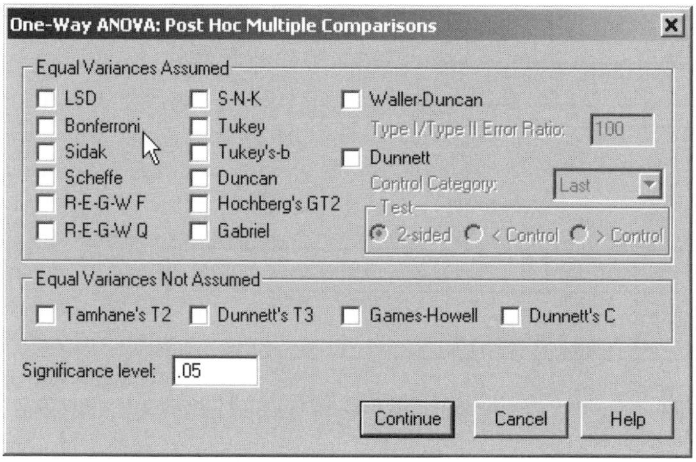

Figure 8.8 The **One-way ANOVA: Post Hoc Multiple Comparisons** box

For example, suppose the data in Table 8.1 and Figure 8.1 appeared as in Figure 8.9. (Compared with the data in Figure 8.1, material A has higher plasticity ratings.)

	plasticy	material
1	18	A
2	19	A
3	20	A
4	19	A
5	21	A
6	16	B
7	13	B
8	12	B
9	11	B
10	13	B
11	14	C
12	10	C
13	11	C
14	13	C
15	15	C

Figure 8.9 The data of Figure 8.1 modified (higher plasticity ratings for material A)

This time, running a one-way ANOVA results in the **Output** shown in Figure 8.10.

Descriptives

plasticity

	N	Mean	Std. Deviation	Std. Error	95% Confidence Interval for Mean Lower Bound	95% Confidence Interval for Mean Upper Bound	Minimum	Maximum
A	5	19.40	1.140	.510	17.98	20.82	18	21
B	5	13.00	1.871	.837	10.68	15.32	11	16
C	5	12.60	2.074	.927	10.03	15.17	10	15
Total	15	15.00	3.606	.931	13.00	17.00	10	21

Test of Homogeneity of Variances

plasticity

Levene Statistic	df1	df2	Sig.
.867	2	12	.445

ANOVA

plasticity

	Sum of Squares	df	Mean Square	F	Sig.
Between Groups	145.600	2	72.800	24.000	.000
Within Groups	36.400	12	3.033		
Total	182.000	14			

Figure 8.10 Output from One-way ANOVA for the data in Figure 8.9 (the value of *F* and its corresponding probability are highlighted)

The null hypothesis can be rejected ($P < 0.0005$). In order to determine which group means differ significantly from each other, we now examine the results of the multiple comparison procedure. In this case the Bonferroni test (which uses *t*-tests to carry out pairwise comparisons between the group means but takes into account the number of tests) has been selected, and part of the results are shown in Figure 8.11.

Post Hoc Tests

Multiple Comparisons

Dependent Variable: plasticity
Bonferroni

(I) MATERIAL	(J) MATERIAL	Mean Difference (I-J)	Std. Error	Sig.	95% Confidence Interval Lower Bound	95% Confidence Interval Upper Bound
A	B	6.40*	1.102	.000	3.34	9.46
	C	6.80*	1.102	.000	3.74	9.86
B	A	-6.40*	1.102	.000	-9.46	-3.34
	C	.40	1.102	1.000	-2.66	3.46
C	A	-6.80*	1.102	.000	-9.86	-3.74
	B	-.40	1.102	1.000	-3.46	2.66

*. The mean difference is significant at the .05 level.

Figure 8.11 Part of the results of a Bonferroni test corresponding to the **Output** in Figure 8.10

From Figure 8.11 it can be seen that group 1 (material A) differs significantly from groups 2 (B) and 3 (C). This is confirmed in the lowest two rows.

NON-PARAMETRIC TESTS

A non-parametric ANOVA should be carried out if the data do not fulfil the criteria for the parametric test given above.

Kruskal–Wallis test

This non-parametric alternative to the parametric test just described requires that the data be measured at least on an ordinal scale. The test statistic (H) is calculated in the same way as the Mann–Whitney test statistic (a non-parametric alternative to the independent samples t-test).

We shall illustrate the use of this test by applying it to the data shown in Table 8.1 and Figure 8.1. The procedure is selected as shown in Figure 8.12.

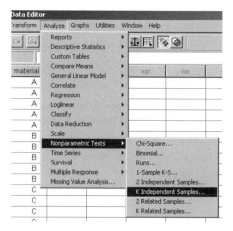

Figure 8.12 Selecting **Nonparametric tests: K Independent Samples**

The resulting box is filled in as shown in Figure 8.13. (Use the **Define Range...** button to enter the minimum and maximum values of the grouping variable.)

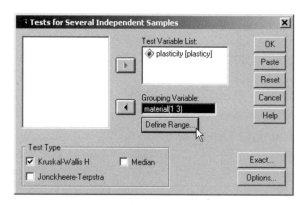

Figure 8.13 The **Tests for Several Independent Samples** box

Click the **Options...** button to obtain the **Options** box (see Figure 8.14), in which **Descriptive** or **Quartiles** can be selected, to give the descriptive statistics for the data.

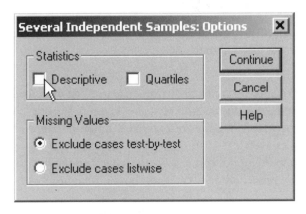

Figure 8.14 The **Tests for Several Independent Samples: Options** box

Click **Continue** to return to the **Tests for Several Independent Samples** box, and then click **OK**. From the **Output** (Figure 8.15) it can be seen that the required probability (corrected for ties) is 0.243 (in this case similar to the parametric test probability of 0.268 found above), which means that the null hypothesis, that the population means are not different, cannot be rejected.

Kruskal-Wallis Test

Ranks

	MATERIAL	N	Mean Rank
plasticity	A	5	10.70
	B	5	6.80
	C	5	6.50
	Total	15	

Test Statistics[a,b]

	plasticity
Chi-Square	2.831
df	2
Asymp. Sig.	.243

a. Kruskal Wallis Test

b. Grouping Variable: MATERIAL

Figure 8.15 Output from Kruskal–Wallis one-way ANOVA

Median test

This non-parametric procedure tests whether two or more samples are drawn from populations with the same median. It uses the chi-square statistic (see Chapter 7) and therefore should not be used if any cell has an expected frequency of less than one or if more than 20% of cells have expected frequencies of less than five. It is carried out by selecting **Median** in the **Tests for Several Independent Samples** box (Figure 8.13) and clicking **OK**.

SIMPLE FACTORIAL ANOVA

Simple factorial ANOVA differs from one-way ANOVA in that it can handle several grouping variables (factors) simultaneously. The criteria that need to be fulfilled for using this test are otherwise essentially the same as those listed under Assumptions in the previous section on One-way ANOVA.

With more than one factor, two types of 'treatment' effects (in ANOVA terminology) can occur:

- *Main effects*, which are the effects of the individual factors.
- An *interaction* between factors; that is, the effects of the factors are mutually dependent.

Procedure

Figure 8.16 shows part of a data file which contains both the plasticity (in arbitrary units) and the method of measuring the plasticity (using one of five methods labelled 1 to 5) of three materials, A to C, for a total of 25 cases.

	plasticy	material	method
1	18	A	1
2	10	A	2
3	20	A	3
4	19	A	4
5	21	A	5
6	16	B	1
7	4	B	2
8	12	B	3
9	11	B	4
10	13	B	5
11	14	C	1
12	11	C	2
13	11	C	3
14	13	C	4
15	15	C	5
16	15	A	1

Figure 8.16 Part of a data file showing both the plasticity and the method of measuring the plasticity (methods 1 to 5) of three materials, A to C, for a total of 25 cases

The corresponding means and standard deviations are obtained by making the selection shown in Figure 8.17.

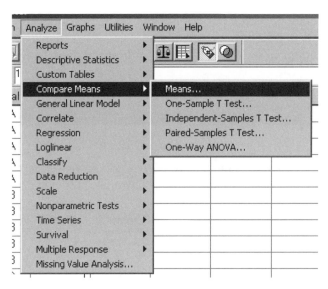

Figure 8.17 Selecting **Compare Means: Means**

In the **Means** box, plasticity is entered as the dependent variable in the **Dependent** list, and material in the **Independent** list, as shown in Figure 8.18.

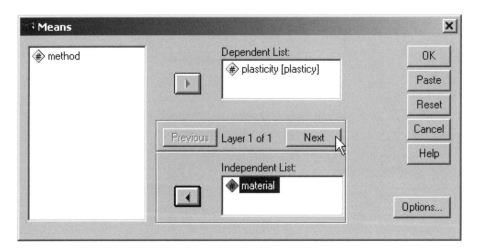

Figure 8.18 The **Means** box

To enter the next layer of classification, click the **Next** button and in the resulting box enter the variable method as shown in Figure 8.19.

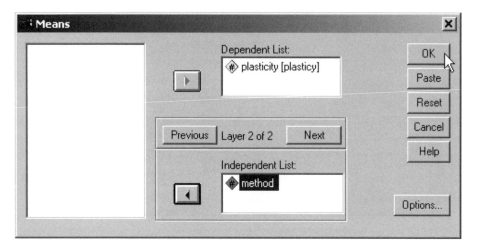

Figure 8.19 Entering layer 2 of 2 in the **Means** box

Click **OK** to obtain the **Output** shown in Figure 8.20. (Notice that a standard deviation is not given when the number of cases in a cell is one.)

Report

plasticity

MATERIAL	METHOD	Mean	N	Std. Deviation
A	1	17.00	2	1.414
	2	7.00	2	4.243
	3	20.00	1	.
	4	19.00	1	.
	5	21.00	1	.
	Total	15.43	7	6.214
B	1	15.00	2	1.414
	2	7.50	2	4.950
	3	12.00	2	.000
	4	11.00	2	.000
	5	13.00	2	.000
	Total	11.70	10	3.129
C	1	14.00	1	.
	2	11.00	1	.
	3	11.00	2	.000
	4	13.00	2	.000
	5	15.00	2	.000
	Total	12.88	8	1.727
Total	1	15.60	5	1.673
	2	8.00	5	3.674
	3	13.20	5	3.834
	4	13.40	5	3.286
	5	15.40	5	3.286
	Total	13.12	25	4.076

Figure 8.20 Output showing summary means and standard deviations of plasticity by levels of material and method

To obtain the means and standard deviations for the variable method, re-open the **Means** box and complete it as shown in Figure 8.21.

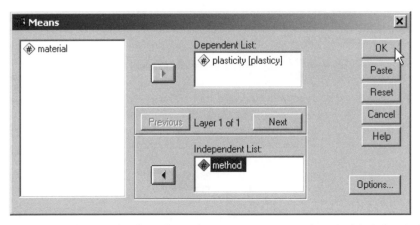

Figure 8.21 The **Means** box completed in order to obtain summary means and standard deviations for levels of the second independent variable (method) of Figs. 8.19 and 8.20

The resulting **Output** is shown in Figure 8.22.

Report

plasticity

METHOD	Mean	N	Std. Deviation
1	15.60	5	1.673
2	8.00	5	3.674
3	13.20	5	3.834
4	13.40	5	3.286
5	15.40	5	3.286
Total	13.12	25	4.076

Figure 8.22 Output showing summary means and standard deviations of plasticity by method

To run a simple factorial ANOVA, use the General Linear model to make the selection shown in Figure 8.23.

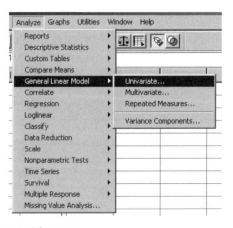

Figure 8.23 Selecting **Simple Factorial ANOVA**

This opens the **Univariate** box, which is completed as shown in Figure 8.24.

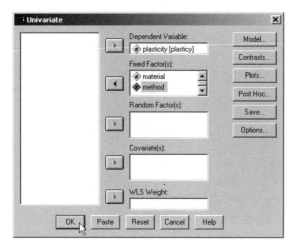

Figure 8.24 The **Simple Factorial ANOVA** box

Clicking **OK** leads to the **Output** shown in Figure 8.25.

Tests of Between-Subjects Effects

Dependent Variable: plasticity

Source	Type III Sum of Squares	df	Mean Square	F	Sig.
Corrected Model	352.140[a]	14	25.153	5.409	.005
Intercept	4264.225	1	4264.225	917.038	.000
MATERIAL	103.721	2	51.861	11.153	.003
METHOD	168.400	4	42.100	9.054	.002
MATERIAL * METHOD	87.873	8	10.984	2.362	.102
Error	46.500	10	4.650		
Total	4702.000	25			
Corrected Total	398.640	24			

a. R Squared = .883 (Adjusted R Squared = .720)

Figure 8.25 Output from Simple Factorial ANOVA (with the values of *F* and their corresponding probabilities highlighted)

From this **Output** it can be seen that there is a significant main effect for the factor material ($P = 0.003$) and for the factor method ($P = 0.002$). These results should be examined in conjunction with the **Outputs** showing the summary means and standard deviations (Figures 8.20 and 8.22), which help explain the findings. The interaction between the two factors is not significant ($P = 0.102$, shown in Figure 8.25).

REPRESENTING INTERACTIONS GRAPHICALLY

To represent interactions graphically, make the selection shown in Figure 8.26.

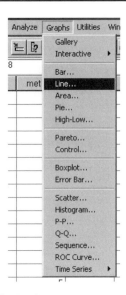

Figure 8.26 Selecting line graphs from the **Graphs** menu

In the next box select **Multiple** for a graph with multiple lines, as shown in Figure 8.27.

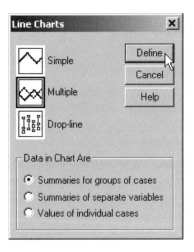

Figure 8.27 Selecting multiple lines in the **Line Charts** box

Click the **Define** button and complete the next box as shown in Figure 8.28. Note that the cell means of the dependent variable, plasticity, will be represented by the lines, while the material has been made the category axis.

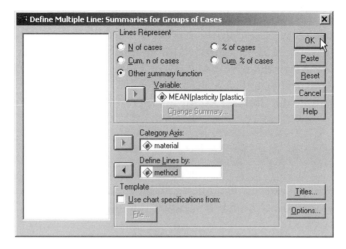

Figure 8.28 The **Define Multiple Lines: Summaries for Groups of Cases** box

Click **OK**. SPSS now produces a graphical representation of the data in the **Output**, as shown in Figure 8.29.

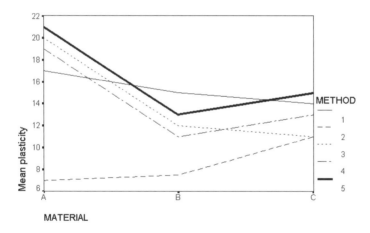

Figure 8.29 Graphical representation of the data of Figure 8.16 (mean plasticity by material and method)

If there were no interaction between the two factors (material and method), the five lines in Figure 8.29 would be parallel. Although this is not the case, they do not strongly deviate from being parallel, in line with the finding that the interaction is not statistically significant.

GENERAL FACTORIAL ANOVA

A covariate is a concomitant variable that is measured in addition to the dependent variable in ANOVA, and that represents an additional, uncontrolled for, source of variation in the dependent variable. For example, in a psychological study of visual perception, age may be a covariate if it has not been controlled for in the experiment. To allow such covariates to be controlled for in an ANOVA that otherwise fulfils the criteria for a simple factorial ANOVA, you can add covariates in the covariate part of the **Univariate** box shown in Figure 8.24. (In versions of SPSS prior to version 10 this is only possible using the **General Factorial ANOVA** menu.)

REPEATED MEASURES ANOVA

This procedure is used to test hypotheses about the means of a dependent variable when the same dependent variable is measured on more than one occasion for each subject.

DEFINITIONS

Between-subjects variables are factors that subdivide the sample into discrete subgroups. Each subject can have only one value for a between-subjects factor.

Within-subjects (repeated measures) variables are factors whose levels are all measured on the same subject.

Mixed (split-plot) design experiments have a mixture of the above two types of variables. Care must be taken in the design of such experiments to reduce carry-over and order effects, for example by counterbalancing.

PARAMETRIC

This is a generalization of the paired samples t-test (see Chapter 6), testing the sources of variation among a group of related dependent variables that represent different measurements of the same attribute.

Mauchly sphericity test and Greenhouse–Geisser epsilon

The criteria that need to be fulfilled to use a repeated measures ANOVA include those listed under the Assumptions subsection in the above section on One-way ANOVA, with the obvious exception that repeated measures are now allowed.

In addition, there is also an assumption that the covariance matrix of the transformed variables has a constant variance on the diagonal and zeros elsewhere. This is tested for using the Mauchly sphericity test. If this test is significant ($P < 0.05$) then the probabilities associated with the values of F from the repeated measures ANOVA should be corrected. This is carried out by multiplying the degrees of freedom (of both the numerator and denominator of the test) by the value of Greenhouse–Geisser epsilon. SPSS gives the value of the latter, and also offers the choice of automatically carrying out this calculation for within-subjects tests, as illustrated in the example that follows.

Procedure

Figure 8.30 shows part of a data file from a study of human visual motion perception, in which sex represents the gender of the subjects, and mot_1 to mot_4 inclusive represent the scores on four successive repeated tests of visual motion. We shall use a repeated measures ANOVA to test whether the visual motion scores vary significantly across the four repeated measures and across gender, and whether there is an interaction between these.

	sex	mot_1	mot_2	mot_3	mot_4
1	Male	15.75	14.03	9.64	12.14
2	Male	15.75	13.24	9.64	11.88
3	Male	6.43	22.27	14.44	7.22
4	Male	18.73	19.28	12.14	26.49
5	Male	5.26	9.92	13.63	8.84
6	Male	19.28	28.88	22.93	16.21
7	Male	10.07	5.25	7.22	7.22
8	Female	25.60	15.75	28.83	17.95

Figure 8.30 Part of a data file from a study of visual motion perception

Repeated measures ANOVA is selected as shown in Figure 8.31.

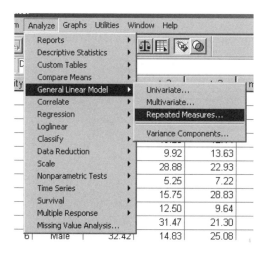

Figure 8.31 Selecting repeated measures ANOVA from the **General Linear Model** menu

This opens the **Repeated Measures Define Factor(s)** box shown in Figure 8.32.

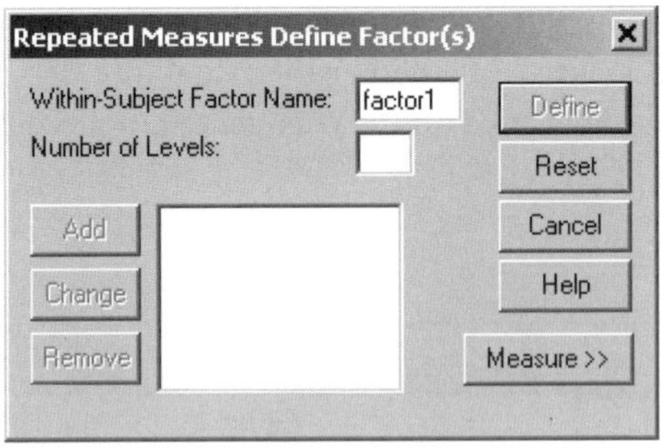

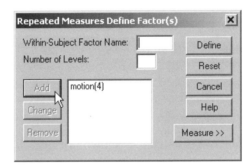

Figure 8.32 The **Repeated Measures Define Factor(s)** box

This is completed as shown in Figure 8.33, from which it can be seen that the name of the within-subject factor (that is, the dependent variable) has been given as motion, and four levels (mot_1 to mot_4) have been entered.

Figure 8.33 Completed **Repeated Measures Define Factor(s)** box

Clicking the **Define** button leads to the **Repeated Measures box,** as shown in Figure 8.34.

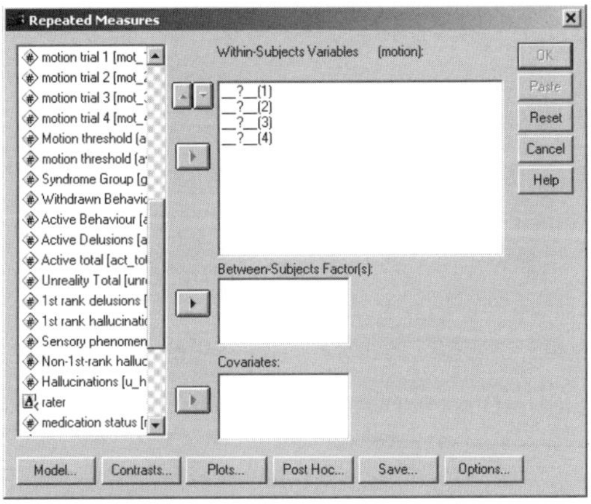

Figure 8.34 The **Repeated Measures** box

This box allows you to specify the tests in which you are interested. The **Within-Subjects Variables** list contains a list of all combinations of factor levels and measures that were defined in the **Define Factors** box. Each combination is preceded by a blank with a question mark in it. The completed **Repeated Measures** box is shown in Figure 8.35, with mot_1 to mot_4 as the four levels of the within-subject factor (dependent variable) motion, and sex as a between-subjects factor.

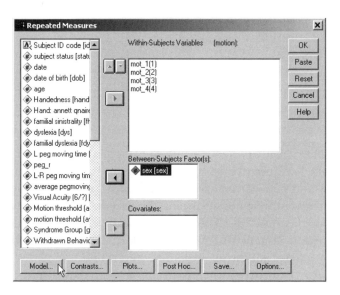

Figure 8.35 Completed **Repeated Measures** box

Click **OK** to obtain the **Output**. Figure 8.36 shows part of the **Output**, containing the results of the Mauchly sphericity test, which is seen to be significant ($P = 0.028$), and the value of Greenhouse–Geisser epsilon (0.741).

Mauchly's Test of Sphericity[b]

Measure: MEASURE_1

Within Subjects Effect	Mauchly's W	Approx. Chi-Square	df	Sig.	Epsilon[a] Greenhouse-Geisser	Huynh-Feldt	Lower-bound
MOTION	.511	12.562	5	.028	.741	.880	.333

Tests the null hypothesis that the error covariance matrix of the orthonormalized transformed dependent variables is proportional to an identity matrix.

a. May be used to adjust the degrees of freedom for the averaged tests of significance. Corrected tests are displayed in the Tests of Within-Subjects Effects table.

b.
Design: Intercept+SEX
Within Subjects Design: MOTION

Figure 8.36 Output showing the results of the Mauchly sphericity test and the value of Greenhouse–Geisser epsilon

A further part of the **Output**, shown in Figure 8.37, contains the results of the ANOVA, based on both uncorrected and corrected degrees of freedom.

Tests of Within-Subjects Effects

Measure: MEASURE_1

Source		Type III Sum of Squares	df	Mean Square	F	Sig.
MOTION	Sphericity Assumed	56.188	3	18.729	1.016	.392
	Greenhouse-Geisser	56.188	2.223	25.270	1.016	.377
	Huynh-Feldt	56.188	2.639	21.289	1.016	.386
	Lower-bound	56.188	1.000	56.188	1.016	.325
MOTION * SEX	Sphericity Assumed	61.555	3	20.518	1.114	.351
	Greenhouse-Geisser	61.555	2.223	27.684	1.114	.342
	Huynh-Feldt	61.555	2.639	23.323	1.114	.347
	Lower-bound	61.555	1.000	61.555	1.114	.304
Error(MOTION)	Sphericity Assumed	1105.566	60	18.426		
	Greenhouse-Geisser	1105.566	44.470	24.861		
	Huynh-Feldt	1105.566	52.785	20.945		
	Lower-bound	1105.566	20.000	55.278		

Figure 8.37 Further **Output** showing the results of the ANOVA

Since the Mauchly sphericity test is significant, the uncorrected degrees of freedom shown in Figure 8.37 need to be multiplied by the value of Greenhouse–Geisser epsilon (0.741) and new corresponding significance values of F calculated. (If the Mauchly sphericity test were not significant, the uncorrected figures could be taken as the final ones for this ANOVA.) This is automatically carried out by SPSS. It can be seen that the corrected significance value is $P = 0.377$. Similarly, the corrected significance value is $P = 0.342$ for the sex by motion interaction.

The results for the between-subjects factor sex are shown further down in the **Output** (see Figure 8.38).

Tests of Between-Subjects Effects

Measure: MEASURE_1
Transformed Variable: Average

Source	Type III Sum of Squares	df	Mean Square	F	Sig.
Intercept	5607.773	1	5607.773	47.839	.000
SEX	100.204	1	100.204	.855	.366
Error	2344.428	20	117.221		

Figure 8.38 Further **Output** showing the between-subjects effects

It can be seen that the corresponding significance value is $P = 0.366$.

Since none of the last three significance values is less than 0.05, there is no evidence that the motion or sex factors have significant main effects. The interaction between motion and sex is also not significant.

NON-PARAMETRIC

Friedman test

This nonparametric test ranks each variable from 1 to k, where k is the number of variables. The mean rank is then calculated for each variable over all the cases. A test statistic is calculated which has an approximately chi-square distribution and which is used to test the null hypothesis that the k related variables come from the same population. This test is therefore suitable for data that are measured on at least an ordinal scale. The following example gives its use for carrying out an ANOVA with ordinal data.

Seven patients undergo a magnetic resonance imaging (MRI) scan of their brains twice each, the first at the onset of a certain brain disorder, and the second six months later. The images are coregistered, with the baseline scans being subtracted from the second scans for each patient. Three different raters are asked independently to rank the resulting MRI results (mri_1 to mri_7) from 1 (highest amount of change) to 7 (least amount of change). The results are shown in Figure 8.39.

	mri_1	mri_2	mri_3	mri_4	mri_5	mri_6	mri_7
1	1	3	5	2	7	6	4
2	3	2	7	4	6	1	5
3	1	5	3	7	4	6	2

Figure 8.39 Data View showing the ranking of MRI results (mri_1 to mri_7) from 1 (highest amount of change) to 7 (least amount of change) by three independent raters

Nonparametric Tests: K Related Samples is selected, as shown in Figure 8.40.

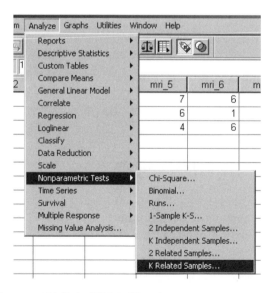

Figure 8.40 Selecting **Nonparametric Tests: K Related Samples**

The resulting box is completed (with the Friedman test selected), as shown in Figure 8.41.

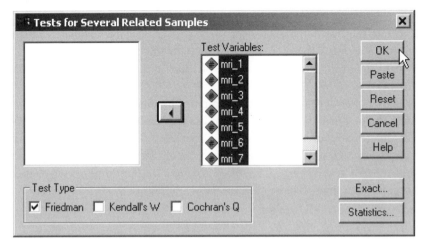

Figure 8.41 The **Tests for Several Related Samples** box with the Friedman test selected

Click on **OK** to obtain the **Output** shown in Figure 8.42.

Friedman Test

Ranks

	Mean Rank
MRI_1	1.67
MRI_2	3.33
MRI_3	5.00
MRI_4	4.33
MRI_5	5.67
MRI_6	4.33
MRI_7	3.67

Test Statistics[a]

N	3
Chi-Square	6.429
df	6
Asymp. Sig.	.377

a. Friedman Test

Figure 8.42 Output showing the results of the Friedman ANOVA

The probability corresponding to the test statistic is $P = 0.377$, and so the rankings of the seven MRI results are not significantly different.

Kendall's W test

This nonparametric test ranks each variable from 1 to k, where k is the number of variables. The mean rank is then calculated for each variable over all the cases. Kendall's W and the corresponding chi-square statistic are then calculated, with ties corrected for. The latter is used to test the null hypothesis that the k related variables come from the same population. This test is therefore suitable for data that are measured on at least an ordinal scale.

W tests for agreement of the rankings by the judges or raters and ranges from 0 (no agreement) to 1 (complete agreement). Each case is assumed to be a judge or rater. Thus Kendall's W test is useful for testing inter-rater reliability.

To determine the value of Kendall's W for the three raters in the previous example (Figure 8.39), complete the **Tests for Several Related Samples** box as shown in Figure 8.43.

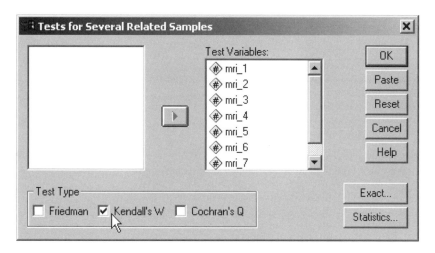

Figure 8.43 The **Tests for Several Related Samples** box with Kendall's W test selected

Clicking **OK** obtains the **Output** shown in Figure 8.44.

Kendall's W Test

Ranks

	Mean Rank
MRI_1	1.67
MRI_2	3.33
MRI_3	5.00
MRI_4	4.33
MRI_5	5.67
MRI_6	4.33
MRI_7	3.67

Test Statistics

N	3
Kendall's W a	.357
Chi-Square	6.429
df	6
Asymp. Sig.	.377

a. Kendall's Coefficient of Concordance

Figure 8.44 Output showing the results of Kendall's W test

The mean rank for each variable is the same as in Figure 8.42, as is the value of chi-square. The value of Kendall's W (for the three raters) is 0.357.

Cochran's Q test

This tests the null hypothesis that the proportion of cases in a particular category is the same for several dichotomous variables. It is suitable for use when there are related samples measured on dichotomous (binary) nominal scales.

Suppose that in the previous example the three raters were asked simply to rate whether they considered significant change had occurred in the MRI results (rated as 1) or not (rated as 0). The corresponding data file is shown in Figure 8.45.

	mri_1	mri_2	mri_3	mri_4	mri_5	mri_6	mri_7
1	1	1	0	1	0	0	0
2	1	1	0	1	0	1	0
3	1	0	1	0	0	0	1

Figure 8.45 Data file showing the dichotomous ratings of MRI results (mri_1 to mri_7) as either 0 (no significant change) or 1 (significant change) by three independent raters

Complete the **Tests for Several Related Samples** box (to select Cochran's Q) as shown in Figure 8.46.

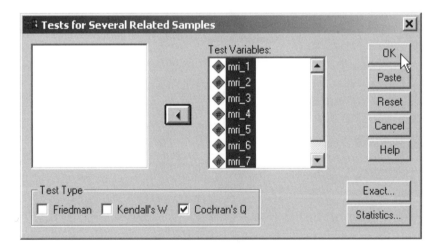

Figure 8.46 The **Tests for Several Related Samples** box with Cochran's Q test selected

Clicking **OK** obtains the **Output** shown in Figure 8.47.

Cochran Test

Frequencies

	Value	
	0	1
MRI_1	0	3
MRI_2	1	2
MRI_3	2	1
MRI_4	1	2
MRI_5	3	0
MRI_6	2	1
MRI_7	2	1

Test Statistics

N	3
Cochran's Q	6.667[a]
df	6
Asymp. Sig.	.353

a. 1 is treated as a success.

Figure 8.47 Output showing the results of Cochran's Q test (significance highlighted)

The probability corresponding to the test statistic is $P = 0.353$, and so the rankings of the seven MRI results are not significantly different.

chapter 9

STATISTICAL ASSOCIATION

In this chapter we are concerned with bivariate data, that is, sets of data involving observations of two variables.

PARAMETRIC TEST

For interval or ratio data that satisfy the normality assumption (see Chapter 4), the Pearson product moment correlation coefficient, often referred to simply as the correlation coefficient, can be used. If the normality assumption is violated, or the data are not interval or ratio, then a nonparametric test should be considered (described later in this chapter).

GRAPHICAL REPRESENTATION

Bivariate data measured on an interval or ratio scale can be represented in the form of scatter diagrams as in Figure 9.1, in which the line of best fit (the linear regression line; see Chapter 10) has been superimposed upon the data.

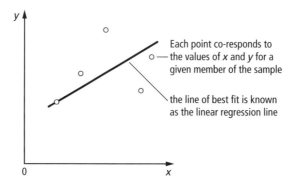

Figure 9.1 A scatter diagram of bivariate data with the linear regression line superimposed. Reproduced from Puri BK (1996) *Statistics for the Health Sciences*, with permission from WB Saunders, London, UK

Finding a statistical association between two variables does not necessarily imply that this association is linear. Graphically, this can be represented by the fact that the line of best fit may not be a straight line. In Figure 9.2, for example, the line of best fit is cubic.

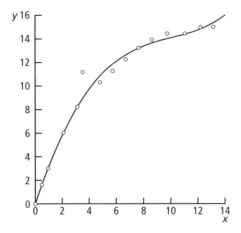

Figure 9.2 A scatter diagram of bivariate data with a cubic line of best fit superimposed. Reproduced from Puri BK (1996) *Statistics for the Health Sciences*, with permission from WB Saunders, London, UK

PEARSON PRODUCT MOMENT CORRELATION COEFFICIENT

This measures the strength of the linear relationship for bivariate data for the two variables. If the two random variables are positively correlated, they tend to increase or decrease together. If they are negatively correlated, one tends to increase as the other decreases.

The value of the Pearson correlation coefficient varies between −1 and 1 inclusive, and does not have any units. Figure 9.3 shows typical scatter diagrams for the range of possible values of the Pearson correlation coefficient, which is denoted by r when obtained from a sample. (The corresponding population correlation coefficient is denoted by ρ.) The range of values is as follows:

- $r = 1$: perfect positive correlation
- $0 < r < 1$: positive though not perfect correlation
- $r = 0$: no correlation
- $-1 < r < 0$: negative though not perfect correlation
- $r = -1$: perfect negative correlation.

SCATTERPLOT OF THE BIVARIATE DATA

It is useful to plot the data in the form of a scatter diagram for the following reasons:

- It provides a useful check on the range in which the correlation coefficient should lie (see Figure 9.3)
- It indicates the presence of any outliers; if these are present their data values should be carefully rechecked in the data file and if correct there, should be checked in the raw data (the correlation coefficient procedure may have to be rerun without the outlier(s))

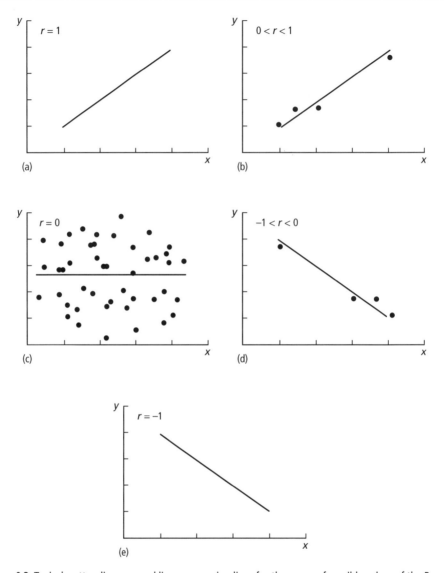

Figure 9.3 Typical scatter diagrams and linear regression lines for the range of possible values of the Pearson product moment correlation coefficient, r. (a) $r = 1$; (b) $0 < r < 1$; (c) $r = 0$; (d) $-1 < r < 0$; (e) $r = -1$. Based on Puri BK (1996) *Statistics for the Health Sciences*, with permission from WB Saunders, London, UK

- It may indicate the shape of the line of best fit, which may not be a straight line but, for example, curved, as in Figure 9.2
- If the line of best fit is not linear, an indication may be given of the type of data transformation that may make it linear

The way in which scatterplots are produced for bivariate data has been explained in Chapter 6.

PROCEDURE

Figure 9.4 shows the data file of the cerebrospinal fluid levels of 5-HIAA (5-hydroxy-indoleacetic acid) and cortisol in 14 untreated patients suffering from depressive disorder. We wish to determine the value of the Pearson product moment correlation coefficient for these two substances in this group of patients.

	hiaa	cortisol
1	100	38
2	52	25
3	50	27
4	48	18
5	124	29
6	167	39
7	147	26
8	112	35
9	102	31
10	148	33
11	70	26
12	58	28
13	97	24
14	120	31

Figure 9.4 Data file of the cerebrospinal fluid levels of 5-HIAA and cortisol in 14 untreated depressed patients (both measured in units of nmol l^{-1} = nM)

The first thing to do is to produce a scatterplot of this set of bivariate data. This is shown in Figure 9.5.

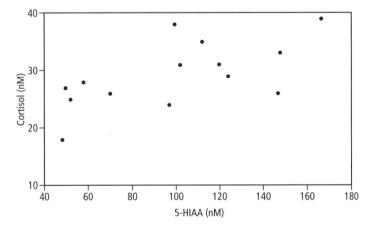

Figure 9.5 Scatterplot of the data file of Figure 9.4

From this scatterplot we can see that the correlation coefficient will lie between 0 and 1 (both exclusive), that there are no obvious outliers, and that it is reasonable to have a line of best fit that is linear.

Check that the normality assumption holds for both variables (see Chapter 4). If it does not, then consider using a nonparametric test (such as the Spearman rank correlation or Kendall's tau-b) instead; these are described later in this chapter.

To determine the actual value of the correlation coefficient, make the selection shown in Figure 9.6.

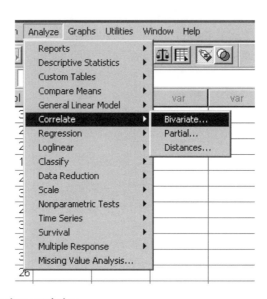

Figure 9.6 Selecting **bivariate correlations**

The resulting **Bivariate Correlations** box is completed as shown in Figure 9.7.

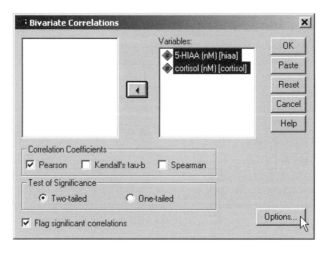

Figure 9.7 The **Bivariate Correlations** box (selecting the Pearson correlation coefficient)

If you would like the values of the means and standard deviations of the two variables to be calculated as well, click the **Options...** button and complete the next box as shown in Figure 9.8.

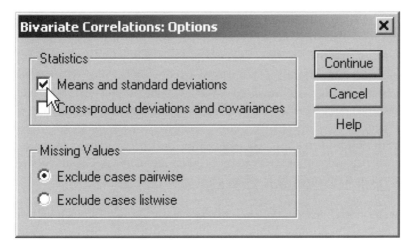

Figure 9.8 The **Bivariate Correlations: Options** box

Click on **Continue** to return to the previous box, and then on **OK** to obtain the **Output** shown in Figure 9.9.

Correlations

Descriptive Statistics

	Mean	Std. Deviation	N
5-HIAA (nM)	99.64	39.521	14
cortisol (nM)	29.29	5.717	14

Correlations

		5-HIAA (nM)	cortisol (nM)
5-HIAA (nM)	Pearson Correlation	1	.630*
	Sig. (2-tailed)	.	.016
	N	14	14
cortisol (nM)	Pearson Correlation	.630*	1
	Sig. (2-tailed)	.016	.
	N	14	14

*. Correlation is significant at the 0.05 level (2-tailed).

Figure 9.9 **Output** showing means, standard deviations and Pearson product moment correlation coefficient for the data shown in Figure 9.4

From this **Output** we can see that for the 5-HIAA the mean level is 99.64 nM with a standard deviation of 39.521 nM. For the cortisol the mean level is 29.29 nM, standard deviation 5.717 nM. The value of the Pearson product moment correlation coefficient is shown as 0.630, based on 14 pairs of cases. This correlation coefficient has an asterisk (*) by it in the **Output** because it is significant at the 0.05 (5%) level, since $P = 0.016$.

NONPARAMETRIC TESTS

ORDINAL DATA

For bivariate data that are measured on at least an ordinal scale (that is, ordinal, interval or ratio), SPSS offers the following two nonparametric tests:

- Spearman's rank correlation. This uses differences between pairs of ranks to give a nonparametric version of the Pearson product moment correlation coefficient.
- Kendall's tau-b is similar to Spearman's rank correlation.

The values of both Spearman's rank correlation and Kendall's tau-b lie in the same range as the Pearson product moment correlation coefficient (between −1 and 1, both inclusive), and their values have similar meanings (a value of 1 implies perfect positive correlation, and so on).

As when determining the Pearson product moment correlation coefficient, it is useful to produce a scatterplot, for the reasons given above.

To illustrate the use of these nonparametric tests, let us suppose the data in Figure 9.4 violated the normality assumption so that we could not use the Pearson correlation coefficient. (As we have already produced a scatterplot (Figure 9.5) and considered its implications, we shall not do so again now.)

Complete the **Bivariate Correlations** box (selected as in Figure 9.6) as shown in Figure 9.10.

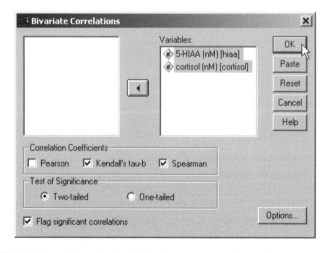

Figure 9.10 The **Bivariate Correlations** box (selecting the nonparametric tests)

Click **OK** to obtain the **Output** shown in Figure 9.11.

Nonparametric Correlations

Correlations

			5-HIAA (nM)	cortisol (nM)
Kendall's tau_b	5-HIAA (nM)	Correlation Coefficient	1.000	.456*
		Sig. (2-tailed)	.	.024
		N	14	14
	cortisol (nM)	Correlation Coefficient	.456*	1.000
		Sig. (2-tailed)	.024	.
		N	14	14
Spearman's rho	5-HIAA (nM)	Correlation Coefficient	1.000	.652*
		Sig. (2-tailed)	.	.012
		N	14	14
	cortisol (nM)	Correlation Coefficient	.652*	1.000
		Sig. (2-tailed)	.012	.
		N	14	14

*. Correlation is significant at the .05 level (2-tailed).

Figure 9.11 Output showing the results of the nonparametric tests for the data file of Figure 9.4

From this **Output** it can be seen that the value of Kendall's tau-b is 0.456 (based on 14 pairs of cases) and that this value is significant (P = 0.024). The value of Spearman's rank correlation is 0.652, which is also significant (P = 0.012).

NOMINAL DATA

Unless the nominal data have a meaningful order (categorical data), no meaning can be attached to a direction of association; rather, the strength of association between two nominal variables is all that can be measured.

SPSS offers the following three measures of association based on the chi-square statistic:

- The phi coefficient. Phi is calculated by dividing the value of chi-square by the sample size and then taking the square root of the result. For 2 × 2 contingency tables SPSS gives phi the same sign as the Pearson correlation coefficient, and its range is from −1 to 1. For tables with more than two rows and/or more than two columns, however, phi can, unfortunately, have a value greater than 1.
- Cramér's V. V is calculated by dividing the value of chi-square by both the sample size and the smaller of the number of rows and columns, and then taking the square root of the result. V always lies between 0 and 1 (inclusive) and can attain a value of 1 for tables of any dimension (unlike the contingency coefficient described next).
- Contingency coefficient. This is calculated by dividing the value of chi-square by the sum of chi-square and the sample size, and then taking the square root of the result. It always lies between 0 and 1 but it is not generally possible to attain the value 1, even for a contingency table showing a perfect relationship. The maximum value depends on the number of rows and columns in the contingency table.

Let us return to the example shown in Figure 7.3, which shows part of a data file from a study on dyslexia, with dyslexic status (normal control or dyslexic) and handedness group (right consistent, mixed preference or left consistent) highlighted. For these two variables we shall determine the values of the above three measures of association.

Follow the steps shown in Figures 7.4 and 7.5 to obtain the **Crosstabs: Statistics** box. This should be completed as shown in Figure 9.12.

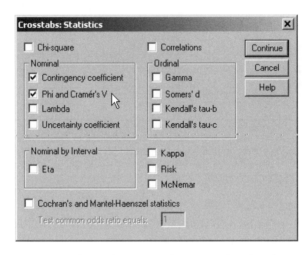

Figure 9.12 The **Crosstabs: Statistics** box with measures of association based on chi-square for nominal data selected

Click **Continue** and then in the next box click **OK** to obtain the **Output** shown in Figure 9.13.

Symmetric Measures

		Value	Approx. Sig.
Nominal by Nominal	Phi	.326	.000
	Cramer's V	.326	.000
	Contingency Coefficient	.310	.000
N of Valid Cases		268	

a. Not assuming the null hypothesis.

b. Using the asymptotic standard error assuming the null hypothesis.

Figure 9.13 Output showing the results of the measures of association based on chi-square for the data shown in Figure 7.3

From this **Output** it can be seen that all three measures of association are significant, and have the following values: phi and Cramér's V both have the value 0.326, while the contingency coefficient has the value 0.310.

chapter 10

LINEAR REGRESSION BETWEEN TWO VARIABLES

In this chapter linear regression between two variables is described. If a scatter diagram shows a non-linear relationship between the two variables (see Chapter 9), then it may be possible to use data transformation (see Chapter 5) to convert this into a linear relationship.

STRAIGHT LINE EQUATION

Any straight line can be represented by means of the equation $y = a + bx$, where y is the dependent variable, a is the intercept on the y-axis, b is the gradient of the line and x is the independent variable. These are shown in Figure 10.1, in which the gradient is positive (and therefore the value of b is positive).

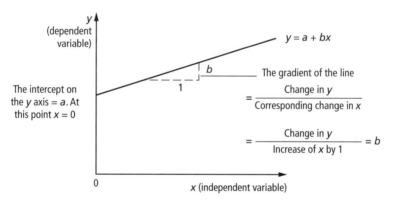

Figure 10.1 The graph of a straight line with positive gradient. Reproduced from Puri BK (1996) *Statistics for the Health Sciences*, with permission from WB Saunders, London, UK

The gradient of the straight line in Figure 10.2 is negative (and therefore the value of b is negative).

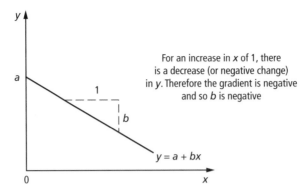

Figure 10.2 The graph of a straight line with negative gradient. Reproduced from Puri BK (1996) *Statistics for the Health Sciences,* with permission from WB Saunders, London, UK

If the gradient of the linear regression line is zero, that is the line is horizontal (and therefore the value of b is zero), there is no linear relationship between the two variables.

LEAST SQUARES METHOD

In order to determine the line of best fit for bivariate data, the least squares method is used. This is shown in Figure 10.3.

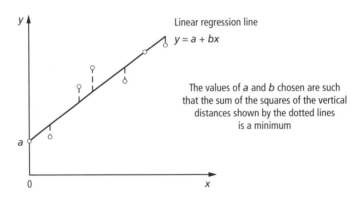

Figure 10.3 The method of least squares to determine the linear regression line. Reproduced from Puri BK (1996) *Statistics for the Health Sciences,* with permission from WB Saunders, London, UK

ASSUMPTIONS

Assumptions made in linear regression include:

● There is no error in the observed values of the independent variable, x.

- For any value of x there is a normal distribution of values of y (see Figure 10.4); these normal distributions for different values of x have the same standard deviation.
- The true mean of each y from these normal distributions (for example y_1 and y_2 in Figure 10.4) lies on the linear regression line.

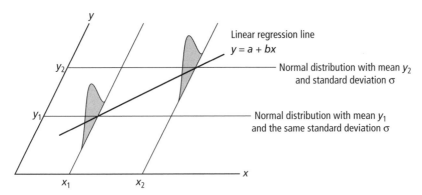

Figure 10.4 Some of the assumptions made in using linear regression. Based on Puri BK and Tyrer P (1992) *Sciences Basic to Psychiatry*, with permission from Churchill Livingstone, Edinburgh, UK

PROCEDURE

As mentioned in the last chapter, it is useful to produce a scatterplot of a set of bivariate data. Amongst other things, this helps to indicate whether or not the shape of the line of best fit is linear, as well as indicating whether there are any outliers (see Chapter 9).

In the previous chapter, Figure 9.4 showed a data file of the cerebrospinal fluid levels of 5-HIAA (5-hydroxyindoleacetic acid) and cortisol in 14 untreated patients suffering from depression. (The Pearson product moment correlation coefficient for these two substances in this group of patients was determined.) We shall determine the equation of the linear regression line for these data, and superimpose this line on the scatterplot of the data (shown in Figure 9.5).

From this scatterplot we can see that there are no obvious outliers and that it is reasonable to have a line of best fit that is linear.

LINEAR REGRESSION EQUATION

Make the selection shown in Figure 10.5.

Complete the resulting linear regression box as shown in Figure 10.6.

Click the **Statistics...** button and in the next box select any additional statistics you require in addition to or instead of the default selections (**Estimates of Regression**

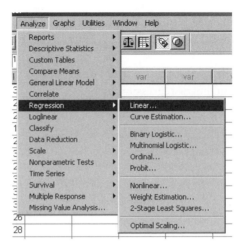

Figure 10.5 Selecting linear regression

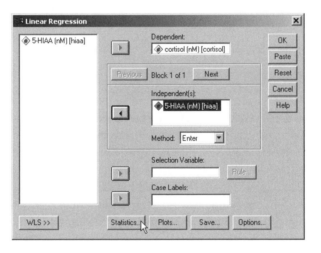

Figure 10.6 The **Linear Regression** box

Coefficients and Model fit). In this case we have additionally selected **Confidence Intervals of the Regression Coefficients** and **Descriptives,** as shown in Figure 10.7.

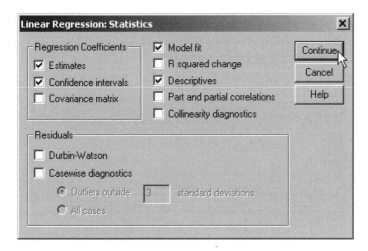

Figure 10.7 The **Linear Regression: Statistics** box

Click **Continue** and then in the previous box click **OK**. The first part of the **Output** contains the descriptive statistics and the correlation coefficient (with one-tailed significance), as shown in Figure 10.8.

Descriptive Statistics

	Mean	Std. Deviation	N
cortisol (nM)	29.29	5.717	14
5-HIAA (nM)	99.64	39.521	14

Correlations

		cortisol (nM)	5-HIAA (nM)
Pearson Correlation	cortisol (nM)	1.000	.630
	5-HIAA (nM)	.630	1.000
Sig. (1-tailed)	cortisol (nM)	.	.008
	5-HIAA (nM)	.008	.
N	cortisol (nM)	14	14
	5-HIAA (nM)	14	14

Figure 10.8 Output from linear regression showing the descriptive statistics and the correlation coefficient with one-tailed significance

It can be seen that the correlation coefficient between the two variables is 0.630, with a one-tailed significance of 0.008, highlighted in Figure 10.8. (Note that in the determination of the correlation coefficient in Chapter 9, the *two*-tailed significance was calculated.) The next part of the **Output** contains the value of R and a linear regression ANOVA, shown in Figure 10.9.

Variables Entered/Removed[b]

Model	Variables Entered	Variables Removed	Method
1	5-HIAA (nM)[a]	.	Enter

a. All requested variables entered.

b. Dependent Variable: cortisol (nM)

Model Summary

Model	R	R Square	Adjusted R Square	Std. Error of the Estimate
1	.630[a]	.396	.346	4.622

a. Predictors: (Constant), 5-HIAA (nM)

ANOVA[b]

Model		Sum of Squares	df	Mean Square	F	Sig.
1	Regression	168.449	1	168.449	7.883	.016[a]
	Residual	256.408	12	21.367		
	Total	424.857	13			

a. Predictors: (Constant), 5-HIAA (nM)

b. Dependent Variable: cortisol (nM)

Figure 10.9 Output from linear regression showing R and a linear regression ANOVA

In the case of the analysis of bivariate data, in which there is just one independent variable, the value of R is the same as that of the Pearson product moment correlation coefficient between the two variables. The number directly next to it, R Square, is the value of the square of the correlation coefficient (r^2). This is also known as the coefficient of determination and is the proportion of the variation in the observed values of y that can be explained by x and therefore by the linear regression line. In this case the proportion is approximately 39.6%. The ANOVA tests whether the relationship between the two variables is linear. This is the case if the value of F is significant (which is the case in Figure 10.9, in which $P = 0.016$) *and* if the scatterplot indicates a linear relationship (which Figure 9.5 does).

The final part of the **Output** gives the variables in the linear regression equation with their confidence intervals and significances (Figure 10.10).

Coefficients[a]

Model		Unstandardized Coefficients		Standardized Coefficients	t	Sig.	95% Confidence Interval for B	
		B	Std. Error	Beta			Lower Bound	Upper Bound
1	(Constant)	20.210	3.460		5.840	.000	12.671	27.750
	5-HIAA (nM)	9.108E-02	.032	.630	2.808	.016	.020	.162

a. Dependent Variable: cortisol (nM)

Figure 10.10 Output from linear regression showing the variables in the equation

Figure 10.10 gives the values for b (0.09108) and a (20.210) in the linear regression equation $y = a + bx$. The standard errors are also given for b (0.032) and a (3.46). The 95% confidence intervals are given for b (0.020 to 0.162) and a (12.671 to 27.750). The significance values for b (0.016) and a (< 0.0005) are clearly both statistically significant.

GRAPH OF LINEAR REGRESSION LINE

Earlier in this book we have shown how to produce a scatterplot of bivariate data (see Chapters 6 and 9). From the **Output** containing this scatterplot, enter the Chart Editor as shown in Figure 10.11 by double-clicking on the scatterplot.

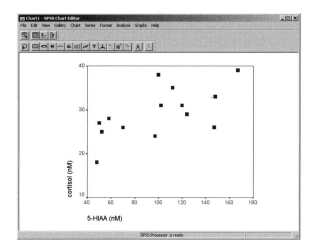

Figure 10.11 The scatterplot in Chart Editor

Make the selection shown in Figure 10.12.

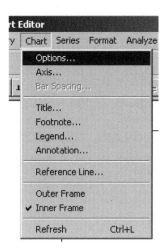

Figure 10.12 Selecting chart options

In the **Fit Line** group in the resulting box, select **Total**, as shown in Figure 10.13.

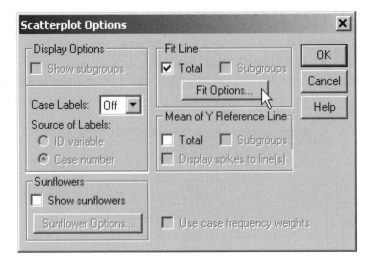

Figure 10.13 The **Scatterplot Options** box

If you wish to check that linear regression is the default setting, click the **Fit Options** box to obtain the **Scatterplot Options: Fit Line** box, shown in Figure 10.14.

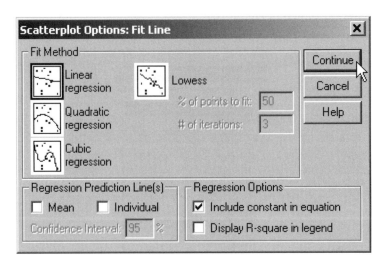

Figure 10.14 The **Scatterplot Options: Fit Line** box

Click **Continue**, and then on returning to the previous box click **OK**. This results in a linear regression being superimposed on the scatterplot, as shown in Figure 10.15.

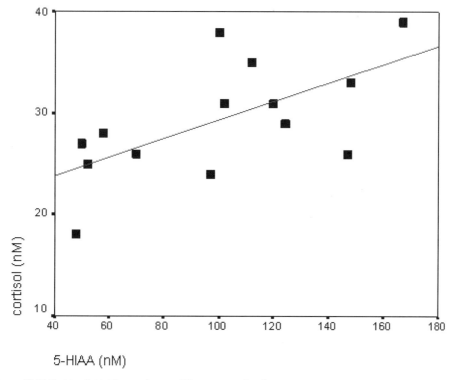

Figure 10.15 Scatterplot with superimposed linear regression line

Note that the intercept of the linear regression line on the left-hand vertical axis is not the same as the value of *a* (20.210). This is because this axis is not the true *y*-axis (*x* = 0), since this chart has started plotting the *x*-axis at the value 40 nM. However, the chart can readily be edited to give a true *y*-axis (*x* = 0) if required.

EXTRAPOLATION AND PREDICTION

The linear regression line equation can be used to predict values of *y* for given values of *x*. However, this should only be carried out for values of *x* lying in the range of *x* used to determine the equation in the first place, and also only if the value of the coefficient of determination, r^2, is not close to zero.

Figure 10.16 illustrates why, when a linear correlation is found between two variables, it must not be assumed that the correlation coefficient, *r*, and the corresponding linear regression line can be extrapolated to include values of *x* and *y* outside the range used in their calculation.

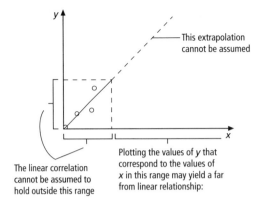

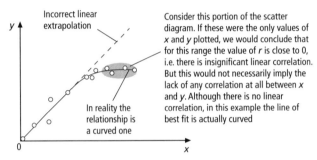

Figure 10.16 Illustration of why extrapolation and prediction may not be valid outside the range used to calculate the correlation coefficient and linear regression equation. Reproduced from Puri BK (1996) *Statistics for the Health Sciences*, with permission from WB Saunders, London, UK

To plot the 95% confidence interval for the predicted means, return to the **Scatterplot Options: Fit Line** box (Figure 10.14) and make the selection shown in Figure 10.17.

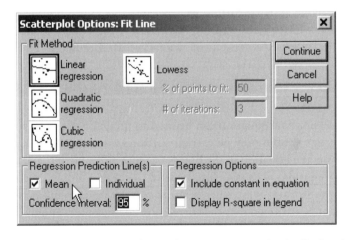

Figure 10.17 The **Scatterplot Options: Fit Line box** – selecting Mean Regression Predication Line(s)

The resulting chart, with the linear regression line and the confidence interval for mean prediction, is shown in Figure 10.18.

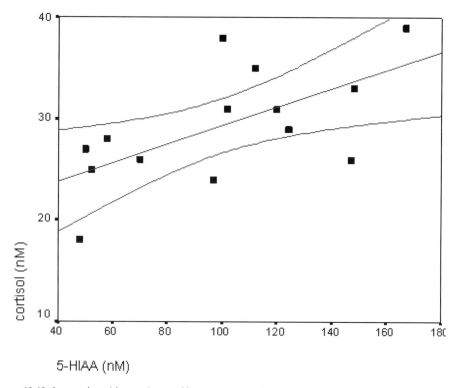

Figure 10.18 Scatterplot with superimposed linear regression line and 95% confidence intervals

APPENDIX

ABS(numexpr) *Numeric* Returns the absolute value of numexpr, which must be numeric.

ANY(test,value[,value,...])) *Logical* Returns 1 or true if the value of test matches any of the subsequent values; returns 0 or false otherwise. It requires two or more arguments.

ARSIN(numexpr) *Numeric* Returns the arcsine, in radians, of numexpr, which must evaluate to a numeric value between -1 and $+1$.

ARTAN(numexpr) *Numeric* Returns the arctangent, in radians, of numexpr, which must be numeric.

CDF.distribution(numexpr,...) *Numeric* Returns the probability that a random variable with a specified distribution would be less than numexpr.

CDFNORM(zvalue) *Numeric* Returns the probability that a random variable with mean 0 and standard deviation 1 would be less than zvalue, which must be numeric.

CFVAR(numexpr,numexpr[,...]) *Numeric* Returns the coefficient of variation (the standard deviation divided by the mean) of its arguments that have valid values. It requires two or more arguments, which must be numeric.

CONCAT(strexpr,strexpr[,...]) *String* Returns a string that is the concatenation of all its arguments, which must evaluate to strings. It requires two or more arguments.

COS(radians) *Numeric* Returns the cosine of a numeric value measured in radians.

CTIME.DAYS(timevalue) *Numeric* Returns the number of days, including fractional days, in timevalue.

CTIME.HOURS(timevalue) *Numeric* Returns the number of hours, including fractional hours, in timevalue.

CTIME.MINUTES(timevalue) *Numeric* Returns the number of minutes, including fractional minutes, in timevalue.

CTIME.SECONDS(timevalue) *Numeric* Returns the number of seconds, including fractional seconds, in timevalue.

DATE.DMY(day,month,year) *Numeric in SPSS date format* Returns a date value corresponding to the indicated day, month, and year. To display this value correctly, assign it a DATE format. The arguments must be integers, with day between 1 and 31, month between 1 and 13, and year a four-digit integer greater than 1582 or a two-digit integer with an assumed prefix of 19.

DATE.MDY(month,day,year) *Numeric in SPSS date format* Returns a date value corresponding to the indicated month, day, and year. To display this value correctly, assign it a DATE format. Arguments are as in the preceding function.

DATE.MOYR(month,year) *Numeric in SPSS date format* Returns a date value corresponding to the indicated month and year. To display this value correctly, assign it a DATE format. The arguments must be integers, with month between 1 and 13, and year a four-digit integer greater than 1582 or a two-digit integer with an assumed prefix of 19.

DATE.QYR(quarter,year) *Numeric in SPSS date format* Returns a date value corresponding to the indicated quarter and year. To display this value correctly, assign it a DATE format. The arguments must be integers, with quarter between 1 and 4, and year a 4-digit integer greater than 1582 or a 2-digit integer with an assumed prefix of 19.

DATE.WKYR(weeknum,year) *Numeric in SPSS date format* Returns a date value corresponding to the indicated weeknum and year. To display this value correctly, assign it a DATE format. The arguments must be integers, with weeknum between 1 and 52, and year a four-digit integer greater than 1582 or a two-digit integer with an assumed prefix of 19.

DATE.YRDAY(year,daynum) *Numeric in SPSS date format* Returns a date value corresponding to the indicated year and daynum. To display this value correctly, assign it a DATE format. The arguments must be integers, with daynum between 1 and 366, and year a four-digit integer greater than 1582 or a two-digit integer with an assumed prefix of 19.

EXP(numexpr) *Numeric* Returns *e* raised to the power numexpr, where numexpr is numeric.

IDF.distribution(prob, ...) *Numeric* Returns the value in a specified distribution with a cumulative probability equal to prob.

INDEX(haystack,needle) *Numeric* Returns an integer that indicates the starting position of the first occurrence of the string needle in the string haystack. Returns 0 if needle does not occur within haystack.

INDEX(haystack,needle,divisor) *Numeric* See the preceding function. The optional third argument divisor is the number of characters used to divide needle into separate strings to be sought. It must be an integer that divides evenly into the length of needle.

LAG(variable) *Numeric or string* Returns the value of variable for the previous case in the data file. Returns system-missing (numeric variables) or blank (string variables) for the first case.

LAG(variable,ncases) *Numeric or string* Returns the value of variable for the case that is ncases earlier in the file. Returns system-missing (numeric variables) or blank (string variables) for the first ncases cases.

LENGTH(strexpr) *Numeric* Returns the length of strexpr, which must be a string expression. This is the defined length, including trailing blanks. To get the length without trailing blanks, use LENGTH(RTRIM(strexpr)).

LG10(numexpr) *Numeric* Returns the logarithm with base 10 of numexpr, which must be numeric and greater than 0.

LG(numexpr) *Numeric* Returns the natural logarithm (base *e*) of numexpr, which must be numeric and greater than 0.

LOWER(strexpr) *String* Returns strexpr with upper-case letters changed to lower case and other characters unchanged.

LPAD(strexpr,length) *String* Returns the string strexpr padded on the left with blanks to extend it to the length given by length, which must be a positive integer between 1 and 255.

LPAD(strexpr,length,char) *String* Identical to LPAD with two arguments, but uses char to pad strexpr on the left. The optional third argument char is a single character within apostrophes, or a string expression that yields a single character.

LTRIM(strexpr) *String* Returns the string strexpr trimmed of any leading blanks.

LTRIM(strexpr,char) *String* Identical to LTRIM with one argument, but trims leading instances of char. The optional second argument char is a single character within apostrophes, or a string expression that yields a single character.

MAX(value,value[,...]) *Numeric or string* Returns the maximum value of its arguments that have valid values. It requires two or more arguments.

MEAN(numexpr,numexpr[,...]) *Numeric* Returns the arithmetic mean of its arguments that have valid values. It requires two or more arguments, which must be numeric.

MIN(value,value[,...]) *Numeric or string* Returns the minimum value of its arguments that have valid values. It requires two or more arguments.

MISSING(variable)) *Logical* Returns 1 or true if variable has a missing value. The argument should be a variable name in the working data file.

MOD(numexpr,modulus) *Numeric* Returns the remainder when numexpr is divided by modulus. Both arguments must be numeric, and the modulus must not be zero.

NCDF.distribution(numexpr, ...) *Numeric* Returns the probability that a random variable with a specified noncentral distribution would be less than numexpr.

NMISS(variable[,...]) *Numeric* Returns a count of the arguments that have missing values. It requires one or more arguments, which should be variable names in the working data file.

NORMAL(stddev) *Numeric* Returns a normally distributed pseudo-random number from a distribution with mean 0 and standard deviation stddev, which must be a positive number. You can repeat the sequence of pseudo-random numbers by setting a Seed in the Preferences dialog box before each sequence.

NUMBER(strexpr,format) *Numeric* Returns the value of the string expression strexpr as a number. The second argument, format, is the numeric format used to read strexpr. Thus if name is an 8-character string containing the character representation of a number, NUMBER(name, f8) is the numeric representation of that number. If the string cannot be read using the format, this function returns system-missing.

NVALID(variable[,...]) *Numeric* Returns a count of the arguments that have valid, non-missing values. It requires one or more arguments, which should be variable names in the working data file.

PROBIT(prob) *Numeric* Returns the value in a standard normal distribution with a cumulative probability equal to prob. The argument prob is a probability greater than 0 and less than 1.

RANGE(test,lo,hi[,lo,hi,...])) *Logical* Returns 1 or true if test is within any of the inclusive range(s) defined by the pairs lo, hi. Arguments must be all numeric or all strings of the same length, and each of the lo, hi pairs must be ordered with lo <= hi.

RINDEX(haystack,needle) *Numeric* Returns an integer than indicates the starting position of the last occurrence of the string needle in the string haystack. Returns 0 if needle does not occur within haystack.

RINDEX(haystack,needle,divisor) *Numeric* See the preceding function. The optional third argument divisor is the number of characters used to divide needle into separate strings to be sought. It must be an integer that divides evenly into the length of needle.

RND(numexpr) *Numeric* Returns the integer that results from rounding numexpr, which must be numeric. Numbers ending in .5 exactly are rounded away from zero.

RPAD(strexpr,length) *String* Returns the string strexpr padded on the right with blanks to extend it to the length given by length, which must be a positive integer between 1 and 255.

RPAD(strexpr,length,char) *String* Identical to RPAD with two arguments, but uses char to pad strexpr on the right. The optional third argument char is a single character within apostrophes, or an expression that yields a single character.

RTRIM(strexpr) *String* Returns the string strexpr trimmed of any trailing blanks. This function is normally used within a larger expression, since strings are padded with trailing blanks upon being assigned to variables.

RTRIM(strexpr,char) *String* Identical to RTRIM with one argument, but trims trailing instances of char. The optional second argument char is a single character within apostrophes, or an expression that yields a single character.

RV.distribution(prob, ...) *Numeric* Returns a random number sampled from a specified distribution.

SD(numexpr,numexpr[,...]) *Numeric* Returns the standard deviation of its arguments that have valid values. It requires at least two arguments, which must be numeric.

SIN(radians) *Numeric* Returns the sine of a numeric value measured in radians.

SQRT(numexpr) *Numeric* Returns the positive square root of numexpr, which must be numeric and not negative.

STRING(numexpr,format) *String* Returns the string that results when numexpr is converted to a string according to format. STRING(-1.5,F5.2) returns the string value '-1.50'. The second argument format must be a format for writing a numeric value.

SUBSTR(strexpr,pos) *String* Returns the substring beginning at position pos of strexpr and running to the end of strexpr.

SUBSTR(strexpr,pos,length) *String* Returns the substring beginning at position pos of strexpr and running for length length.

SUM(numexpr,numexpr[,...]) *Numeric* Returns the sum of its arguments that have valid values. It requires two or more arguments, which must be numeric.

SYSMIS(numvar)) *Logical* Returns 1 or true if the value of numvar is system-missing. The argument numvar must be the name of a numeric variable in the working data file.

TIME.DAYS(days) *Numeric in SPSS time-interval format* Returns a time interval corresponding to the indicated number of days. To display this value correctly, assign it a TIME format. The argument must be numeric.

TIME.HMS(hours,min,sec) *Numeric in SPSS time-interval format* Returns a time interval corresponding to the indicated number of hours, min, and sec. To display this value correctly, assign it a TIME format. The arguments must be integers no greater than 24, 60, and 60, respectively, except that the first nonzero argument can exceed its limit, and the last argument can have a fractional part.

TRUNC(numexpr) *Numeric* Returns the value of numexpr truncated to an integer (toward zero).

UNIFORM(max) *Numeric* Returns a uniformly distributed pseudo-random number between 0 and the argument max, which must be numeric (but can be negative). You can repeat the sequence of pseudo-random numbers by setting the same Random Number Seed before each sequence.

UPCAS(strexpr) *String* Returns strexpr with lower-case letters changed to upper case and other characters unchanged.

VALUE(variable) *Numeric or string* Returns the value of variable, ignoring user missing-value definitions for variable, which must be a variable name in the working data file.

VARIANCE(numexpr,numexpr[,...]) *Numeric* Returns the variance of its arguments that have valid values. It requires at least two arguments, which must be numeric.

XDATE.DATE(datevalue) *Numeric in SPSS date format* Returns the date portion from a numeric value in SPSS date format.

XDATE.HOUR(datevalue) *Numeric* Returns the hour (an integer between 0 and 23) from a numeric value in SPSS date format.

XDATE.JDAY(datevalue) *Numeric* Returns the day of the year (an integer between 1 and 366) from a numeric value in SPSS date format.

XDATE.MDAY(datevalue) *Numeric* Returns the day of the month (an integer between 1 and 31) from a numeric value in SPSS date format.

XDATE.MINUTE(datevalue) *Numeric* Returns the minute (an integer between 0 and 59) from a numeric value in SPSS date format.

XDATE.MONTH(datevalue) *Numeric* Returns the month (an integer between 1 and 12) from a numeric value in SPSS date format.

XDATE.QUARTER(datevalue) *Numeric* Returns the quarter of the year (an integer between 1 and 4) from a numeric value in SPSS date format.

XDATE.SECOND(datevalue) *Numeric* Returns the second (a number between 0 and 60) from a numeric value in SPSS date format.

XDATE.TDAY(timevalue) *Numeric* Returns the number of whole days (as an integer) from a numeric value in SPSS time-interval format.

XDATE.TIME(datevalue) *Numeric in SPSS time-interval format, representing the number of seconds since midnight* Returns the time of day from a numeric value in SPSS date format.

XDATE.WEEK(datevalue) *Numeric* Returns the week number (an integer between 1 and 53) from a numeric value in SPSS date format.

XDATE.WKDAY(datevalue) *Numeric* Returns the day-of-week number (an integer between 1, Sunday, and 7, Saturday) from a numeric value in SPSS date format.

XDATE.YEAR(datevalue) *Numeric* Returns the year (as a four-digit integer) from a numeric value in SPSS date format.

YRMODA(year,month,day) *Numeric* Returns the number of days from October 15, 1582 to the date represented by the arguments year, month, and day, which must be integers that form a valid date since October 15, 1582. Two-digit values of year are prefixed with 19.

INDEX